HEALTHY TEETH FOR KiDS

HEALTHY TEETH *FOR* KiDS

A Preventive Program: From Pre-birth Through the Teens

Jerome S. Mittelman, D.D.S., F.A.P.M.
Beverly D. Mittelman, B.S., C.N.C.
Jean Barilla, B.A., B.S., M.S.

TWIN STREAMS
Kensington Publishing Corp.
http://www.kensingtonbooks.com

KENSINGTON BOOKS are published by

Kensington Publishing Corp.
850 Third Avenue
New York, NY 10022

All Kensington titles, imprints and distributed lines are available at special quantity discounts for bulk purchases for sales promotion, premiums, fund-raising, educational or institutional use.

Special book excerpts or customized printings can also be created to fit specific needs. For details, write or phone the office of the Kensington Special Sales Manager: Kensington Publishing Corp., 850 Third Avenue, New York, NY 10022. Attn. Special Sales Department. Phone: 1-800-221-2647.

ISBN 1-57566-611-1

First Printing: June, 2001
10 9 8 7 6 5 4 3 2 1

Printed in the United States of America

*To Weston A. Price, D.D.S., nutrition
researcher and pioneer, whose studies
demonstrated that dental disease is a disease
of civilization, and to Emanuel Cheraskin,
M.D., D.D.S., whose research confirms and
continues Price's work.*

—J. M. and B. M.

*To all the children, present and future,
who deserve to have healthy bodies and
beautiful smiles.*

—J. B.

Acknowledgments

Our thanks to William G. Crook, M.D., who has been so instrumental in making us aware of the yeast connection and whose advice to Lee Heiman at Kensington led to this book becoming a reality. Our thanks, too, to our coauthor, Jean Barilla, for making some complicated concepts reader-friendly.

—J. M. and B. M.

I thank my coauthors Jerry and Bev Mittelman for their enthusiastic support of my efforts to make this book scientifically accurate and a good reading experience. Thanks also to Kensington's Lee Heiman who convinced me that parents everywhere needed this book, and to my editor, Claire Gerus, for her good advice and kind words. I sincerely thank my husband, George Barilla, for his love and understanding during this endeavor.

—J. B.

Contents

Preface

The three of us—a dentist, a nutritionist, and a medical educator—got together one day and decided to write this book. Why? Because no other book offers this step-by-step program to assure your child of healthy teeth.

We begin when your child is a dream in your heart and take you through a healthy pregnancy and childbirth, from infancy through toddler time and right up to the teen years.

Jerome and Beverly Mittelman:
In our experience, most dentists are preoccupied with "crisis dental care." Almost everything dentists do is repair work—restoring a breakdown in the mouth, repairing cavities with fillings, doing root canal therapy, extractions, crowns, eventually bridges.

Unlike most dentists, we believe in "preventive" dentistry, and when possible, we like to start with "primary" prevention (which actually starts before birth). The more you understand and pay attention to prevention, the fewer dental repairs your children will need later on. That's what this book is about—primary prevention.

In this book we'll tell you how to help your children have bright, strong, healthy teeth; firm, pink gums; a great smile—and see the dentist for no more than checkups. Our motto is: *There's no dentistry as good as "no dentistry"!*

We often told our patients, "The more you listen to us, the less you'll need us." A shiny fork hung down from the ceiling in each room of our office, suspended by dental floss. When patients asked what those forks were doing there, our staff pointed out that if people kept their teeth as clean as they kept their silverware, they wouldn't need us.

Outside the treatment room was a sign that said "Repairs." An arrow pointing to the other rooms said "Prevention." Someday, we hope, that the "Repairs" sign will come down for good. We believe that truly good dentistry tries to do away with the need for these services.

One of the "Prevention" rooms was the dental hygienist's room. Hygienists play a vital role in preventing dental disease in three ways: first, by showing patients how to get a really healthy mouth; second, by scaling and polishing teeth to create a smooth surface that won't trap plaque, and so gums can heal; third, to help the dentist keep watch on the health of the patient's mouth.

In addition to these important activities, our hygienist monitored the patients' nutrition. One question she routinely asked was, "What did you have for breakfast?" If protein was not on the breakfast menu, there was a good chance that the patient's immune system and dental health were not at full strength. A patient's breakfast food choices gave her a clue to the rest of the diet.

Patients were also asked, "Are you taking any nutritional supplements?" If the answer was "no", the hygienist would give the patient information on the importance of supplements to the health of the gums.

Our hygienist also did a simple vitamin C level test by putting a drop of harmless dye on the patient's tongue. If it took more than 15 seconds for the cells on the surface of the tongue to decolorize the dye, she would advise the patient that he or she needed to take more vitamin C. Then she would check the saliva to see whether it was too acidic by placing a little saliva on a strip of pH test paper. High acidity would suggest that the patient was eating too many refined carbohydrates, which is an important factor in gum disease as well as the development of cavities.

In another room, Beverly offered nutrition counseling, gave patients practical suggestions to improve their diets, and recommended supplements. She also did myofunctional therapy to retrain incorrect swallowing patterns with special exercises. It's surprising how common these patterns are and how many difficulties they can cause, including orthodontic problems and irregularities in the bite, which can lead to TMJ disorder and pain in the neck and head.

Our efforts to enlighten our patients continued in the reception room. We had a rack of spice jars filled with the amount of sugar that would be found in the food on each label:

1 tbsp jam or jelly	3 tsp
1 cup chocolate milk	6 tsp
1 doughnut	4 tsp
1 can soda	9 tsp
1 stick chewing gum	½ tsp

Hanging down from the rack on a string was an apothecary jar with 18 teaspoons of sugar, representing a slice of pie with ice cream.

We also offered a lending library of books on nutrition, and scrapbooks of reprints of articles on oral health and nutrition from magazines. In total, we were a "full-service" establishment! Even after the patients left the office, we continued to stay in touch by sending out a quarterly newsletter on preventive dentistry, to let them know the latest dental care news. Now, in this book, we've taken the best of what we gave our patients, and we offer it to our readers.

Jean Barilla:

As a health educator, I have spent years teaching people what makes a healthy body. *Healthy cells make healthy bodies.* Good nutrition produces healthy cells. If you feed your cells the nutrients they need to be the best they can be, the whole body will be healthy, including the cells that will form your child's teeth.

A cell that doesn't get good nourishment may survive, but it will be smaller, won't work as well at its intended job, and will die sooner. The teeth, liver, heart, brain, or other body organ that these cells will form will also wear out early. Good nutrition can prevent this from happening.

At the moment of conception, all the cells in your child's body begin to grow and develop. Will these cells find themselves in an environment where every nutrient they need is available in the right amount? Although I told my children that I could hear their cells "crying out for broccoli," the truth is that cells can't tell you what they need.

This book, however, will show you how you can feed your child the nutrients his or her cells need for healthy teeth, as well as a healthy body. Thanks to years of study, I was able to confer a wonderful legacy on my two children: they have almost perfect teeth, and my grandchildren received an excellent dietary start—even before conception. Today, all three of my grandchildren, aged 8, 11, and 13, have cavity-free teeth. I'd like the same for you and your children and grandchildren. So I invite you to read on.

Introduction

An old Japanese custom considers a baby to be a year old on the day of its birth. By the time the umbilical cord is tied, much has already happened to the newborn. Anything that affected the mother during pregnancy—disease and nutritional deficiencies, injury, radiation or drug exposure, genetic influences, and even emotional reactions—may interfere with the normal growth and development of her baby. Thus, at birth, far from having a "clean slate," an infant comes into the world with all its mother's experiences.

Therefore, preventing problems before they occur—primary prevention—really starts long before your child cuts his or her first tooth. In fact, you'll begin to ensure that your child will have healthy, straight teeth when you begin planning to have that child—months before conception. Your nutrition habits and health are crucial; even the father's health plays an important role in healthy development. Key nutrients must be present at the moment that sperm meets egg for optimal development of your baby's body—including his or her future teeth.

Science shows us that every cell, tissue, and organ in your baby's body can be changed before birth by any one of a number of physical, chemical, microbial, or even psychological challenges. Even morning sickness must be prevented so that a mother is well nourished. In this book, we offer solutions to relieve morning sickness. We also explain the vital role of breast feeding in the development of the jaws, the teeth, and even the face. With this knowledge and a host of other practical and often fascinating recommendations, you will have the power to engineer your child's dental future. Just like any other body part, teeth and gums are tissues that require the best environment in which to flourish. The health of your child's mouth and teeth, as you will learn in this book, affects his or her entire body, including the heart and the immune system.

This book presents a truly holistic approach to giving your child the best start for a lifelong healthy mouth—and body. The importance of diet, knowing when supplements are needed, and learning to avoid environmental pollutants are all part of the equation. The other side of the prevention coin is secondary prevention: catching problems early—stopping them in their tracks before they become catastrophes. Then, by making sure these problems never recur, your child will enjoy the lasting benefits of healthy teeth and a dazzling smile. This book will help you:

- Select the right family dentist
- Understand the vital role of breast feeding—and its alternatives
- Curb thumb sucking, a threat to oral health
- Choose the best toothpaste, toothbrush, floss, and mouthwash
- Use the pacifier as an oral exerciser
- Understand why brushing immediately after eating sugar is too late
- Find ways to keep sugar away from children
- Become familiar with herbs, flower remedies, and homeopathic remedies that can ease dental problems
- Avoid dental procedures, materials, and drugs that may have adverse effects on your children

Other key information in this book includes:

- Knowing when to take your child for that first dental visit
- The best oral hygiene methods from birth through the toddler years
- The hazards of some common dental procedures
- Newer, safer dental techniques and materials

Remember, the advice presented here can guide you and your child for a lifetime. The rewards will be many: self-confidence, good health, financial savings, and an excellent start for the next generation. Consider dental health a far-reaching insurance policy—one that guarantees that you and your children will be the beneficiaries!

Jerome Mittelman
Beverly Mittelman
Jean Barilla

CHAPTER 1

Pregnancy: When Prevention Begins

Were they called upon to name the most important factor in contributing to the health development of the human [fetus], most authorities would unhesitantly declare for the good nutrition status of the mother.

—Ashley Montagu, Ph.D.,
Prenatal Influences

Preparing for Pregnancy

Dr. Westin Price, a nutrition pioneer and dentist, traveled the world in the early twentieth century looking for the cause of the rampant dental disease he saw in "civilized countries." In isolated places like South America, Polynesia, and the Far North, he found people with perfect teeth and no gum disease. It wasn't good genes that protected them—it was good nutrition. They ate what their ancestors had eaten and were healthy. When their diets became "civilized," they lost their teeth and their health.

Conceiving, carrying, and giving birth are all part of a biological process. A set of very specific rules must be followed and special conditions met to ensure success. The different stages in development follow a plan that is written in the genetic code of every cell. Like a musical concert, it can easily lose its harmony if all the instruments do not work properly. The quality of growth conditions that you provide for your baby determines whether each cell will realize its full potential—whether there will be good development, abnormal development, or no development at all. Make no mistake—what you do counts!

When do you start to prepare for pregnancy and provide the best growth conditions for your baby? Is the right time after you conceive, a month before conception, 3 months before, or as soon as you decide that someday you will become a mother or a father? The sooner you start, the higher the probability that you will give a new life the best chance.

If your goal is preventing dental disease and ensuring the best tooth development for your baby, what better way to do this than to ensure that the *whole baby* is healthy? Whether your baby is in the planning stage or already a reality, you *can* make a difference. Each positive step you take, each negative step you avoid, count toward achieving the goal of a healthy baby. As a mother, your body is the source of your baby's life and will be the first environment that your baby lives in. Let's make sure it is the best environment possible.

For Both Parents

It's a good idea for both you and your mate to visit the doctor, particularly if you have had major health problems or problems with a previous pregnancy. If there *was* a problem with a pregnancy, you and your doctor can try to identify what went wrong and possible ways to avoid problems. It is easier to discuss these matters when you are not pregnant.

If you don't already know, each of you should ask your parents whether there is a family history of problem pregnancies or birth defects. A family history may identify any genetic risks. If there is a risk, both parents can get genetic counseling and tests to identify genetic abnormalities.

If you are in the pregnancy-planning stages, now is the time to stop using hormonal birth control. If you were taking birth control pills, stop and use other forms of contraception until you are ready to conceive. Let your body regain its normal menstrual rhythm. Most important, you need to restore nutrients that can be destroyed by contraceptive pills, such as vitamin C, vitamin E, and the B vitamins, especially folic acid. Many women who have been on birth control pills wisely start taking prenatal vitamins 2 or 3 months before they attempt to conceive. As you will see later, correcting a folic acid deficiency is the single best thing you can do to give your baby lifelong health. And don't forget that the father-to-be needs good nutrition, too.

In addition to eating a healthy diet, common sense will tell you, for your baby's sake, to avoid smoking, drinking alcohol, caffeine in excess, or taking street drugs—none of these have ever been proved safe for your baby. Cocaine, for example, causes premature birth and tears in the placenta that can end a pregnancy. Most, if not all, illegal drugs will cross the placenta and harm or even kill your baby. Even if the baby's father takes drugs, your baby can have birth defects.

Alcohol is a known cause of birth defects, with babies being born smaller, with small heads and mental defects. No one knows whether small amounts of alcohol cause damage, because a woman who drinks will never know if her baby could have been smarter if she didn't drink.

Tobacco is the leading preventable cause of low birth weight. Smoking while pregnant is like putting your baby in front of the tail pipe of your car. Tobacco smoke contains carbon monoxide like car exhaust. When the baby's heart and blood vessels are forming, carbon monoxide can cause defects that can be major and cause death or require surgery after birth. Some defects won't be noticed until your child is 20 or 30 years old—perhaps dying suddenly from a burst blood vessel made defective by exposure to cigarette smoke.

Other things to avoid are exposure to solvents (dry cleaning fluids, paints, photographic liquids, and furniture refinishers), traffic fumes, and strong house cleaning products. Be especially aware that pesticides and insecticides used early in pregnancy can result in severe brain and spinal defects in babies.

When both parents-to-be know about the increased pregnancy risks (to both mother and baby), they have a choice. They can choose to accept the risks, be careful and modify or change the risks, or choose to avoid having children. Given the world we live in, it is impossible to avoid every harmful substance in the environment, but every positive step counts toward a brighter future for your baby.

The Father's Health

Most people still think that only the mother has to worry about what she eats and what type of environmental exposure is present before conception. However, it takes two parents to make a healthy baby. To begin with, male fertility cannot be taken for granted. Many factors can affect the number, strength, and vitality of sperm and even the genetic material they carry. In fact, for some reason, men's sperm counts worldwide have been dropping over the last 50 years.

Chemical pollution may be to blame. Some toxic chemicals, especially insecticides, are known to be very damaging to sperm.

Smoking and sexually transmitted diseases are also making men sterile. According to Dr. David Savitz of the School of Public Health at the University of North Carolina, Chapel Hill, men should protect themselves from even casual exposure to lead, alcohol, cigarette smoke, illicit drugs, herbicides, radiation, and some industrial solvents. Toxin-induced damage to sperm may increase the risk of children with birth defects, childhood cancer, and subtle behavioral problems. A father's exposure to chemicals also increases the risk of miscarriage.

In addition, men who smoke are more likely to have children with a cleft lip and palate, and both cigarette smoking and alcohol use by fathers increase the risk of the baby's having a heart defect.

The Prospective Mother's Health

Before she becomes pregnant, a woman should check her health and nutrition status to give her future baby the best start in life. Vaccinations should be up to date because it is dangerous (for the baby) to get shots once a woman is pregnant. This evaluation of health and nutrition should include dental health. As we will see, an unhealthy mouth will affect a woman's whole body, including her unborn baby.

It is important not to be underweight or overweight during pregnancy. Underweight women tend to have smaller babies; these babies have more problems during labor and after delivery. Overweight women are more likely to develop high blood pressure or diabetes during pregnancy. Do *not* diet during pregnancy! It is one of the worst things you can do to your baby. Do not even diet while you are trying to become pregnant. Dieting may deprive your body of key nutrients necessary for conception, and such deficiencies will affect the early normal development of your baby.

The Institute of Medicine, a part of the National Academy of Sciences in Washington, D.C., recommends that underweight women gain as much as 40 pounds during pregnancy, while overweight women should limit their weight increases to 25 pounds.

Medical Problems

If you have diabetes, make sure it is being treated. Although women with insulin-dependent diabetes have a higher risk of miscarriage and of having a baby with a birth defect, if the blood sugar is controlled before and during pregnancy, chances for delivering a healthy baby are excellent. If you have high blood pressure or any other disease, you will need to work out a plan for a safe pregnancy with your doctor. There are natural alternatives to medications for high blood pressure.

Dental Health

Can your dental health affect the outcome of your pregnancy? Current research says "yes." Ten percent of all U.S. births (about 250,000) are premature, low-birth-weight deliveries. Low-birth-weight infants are more likely to die immediately after birth, and survivors may have more neurological problems, respiratory problems, and birth defects.

Periodontal (gum) disease can actually cause premature births. Researcher and periodontist Dr. Steven Offenbacher at the University of North Carolina Hospital found that mothers with periodontal disease had a more than seven times higher risk of premature, low-birth-weight babies. According to Dr. Offenbacher, gum infection in the mother can cause a buildup of *endotoxins,* harmful substances that can get into the bloodstream and reach the unborn child. These endotoxins can cause an increase in inflammation-causing compounds known to be associated with premature birth.

Gum infection toxins can also prevent the body's defenders, the white blood cells, from fighting infection in other parts of a mother's body. The suspected role of gum infections in premature births was confirmed when the bacterium *Fusobacterium nucleatum* was found in the uteruses of women who delivered early. This bacterium is the most frequent type found in *amniotic fluid* (the water surrounding the baby) in women who went into labor early. Surprisingly, this bacterium is not found in the vagina. However, it is commonly found in the mouth and may have spread to amniotic fluid through the blood.

It is now believed that a woman who begins pregnancy with periodontal disease will see it worsen during pregnancy because of hormonal changes and the greater demand by the body for nutrients. However, women who have no periodontal disease, maintain good oral hygiene, and get regular dental care should not expect gum inflammation or an increase in symptoms.

Safe Dental Care

Pregnant women do have a special need for good oral hygiene, but tooth decay results from repeated acid attacks on tooth enamel, not from repeated pregnancies. Gingivitis, a condition of irritated gums that have a tendency to bleed, may occur more often due to a rise in estrogen levels. This can be prevented by having plaque (see chapter 5) removed by a dental hygienist and by eating properly—having protein for breakfast, eliminating refined carbohydrates (sugar), and getting enough vitamins E and C (with bioflavonoids), coenzyme Q_{10} (which is now being added to toothpaste), zinc, and beta-carotene to help increase resistance to infection.

Continue your regular dental visits throughout pregnancy to ensure the best possible care. These visits should include an oral examination (including screening for oral cancer), X-rays if necessary, and a dental cleaning. During the cleaning the dentist will remove dental plaque, then polish your teeth. If it has been a while since your last cleaning, you may need deeper scaling (scraping) to remove tartar deep below the gum line where a toothbrush or floss won't reach. For such procedures, the dentist will usually numb the area. Natural pain relievers should be requested.

Ideally, all major dental work should be done before you become pregnant. It is safe, however, to have dental work done during pregnancy if precautions are followed, as recommended by the American Dental Association (ADA). Dentists will want to wait to schedule treatment during the second trimester—from the fourth to the sixth month. By this time all the major organs are formed in the baby.

Some women may be more anxious, more nervous, or more subject to gagging during the first few months of pregnancy, especially if there are problems with morning sickness. In the final months of pregnancy, you may not be comfortable during a dental procedure, and if you have a history of premature birth, you should avoid dental treatment during this time. If dental X-rays are necessary, be sure a leaded apron is used to prevent exposure to the developing baby. New types of X-ray machines decrease radiation exposure. We will discuss these in a later chapter.

If it is necessary to use drugs or anesthetics during treatment, your dentist should consult with your physician beforehand and make sure there are no side effects that would harm the baby. Although there are no natural or completely safe anesthetics, there are other methods for blocking pain. There is an electric stimulation system that controls pain for most dental procedures without needles, chemicals, or numbness. Instead, an electric current blocks pain transmission in the nerves of the mouth. Hypnosis and dental acupuncture are also used to stop pain.

A Tooth Lost for Every Pregnancy: Fact or Fiction?

It is not true that "a tooth is lost for every pregnancy." In fact, the baby's calcium needs are supplied by nutrients stored in the mother's body—not by her teeth! Tooth decay is the result of repeated acid attacks on tooth enamel from too many carbohydrates eaten too often. If plaque is allowed to remain on teeth, decay and eventual tooth loss can result.

A Hidden Danger to Your Baby: A Mouth Full of Poison

You may be hurting your unborn child without even knowing it. The majority of women of childbearing age (and men as well) have filling material in their teeth that contains a poison. Those nice shiny "silver" fillings are, in fact, not made of silver. They are called *silver amalgam fillings,* but the main ingredient (45–50%) is the toxic metal mercury. Silver accounts for only about 33% of the finished amalgam. The balance can be varying amounts of zinc, copper, and tin. But it is the mercury that we must worry about.

Mercury is one of the most toxic elements on earth, and we will discuss it in more detail in chapter 11. Although it was clearly shown as early as 1926 that mercury vapor is released from mercury amalgam dental fillings, the dental profession chose to ignore this fact. Dentists have always been taught that once mercury has been combined into the filling material, it remains "locked in" and can't come out. But there is much evidence showing that it does come out. It is simple for scientists to determine how much mercury has escaped from any given filling. Since new fillings have 50% mercury, old fillings can be analyzed. If 40% is left, then 10% was lost as vapor or particles from abrasion or corrosion that were most likely swallowed. Mercury tends to collect in certain organs of the body and stay there for different lengths of time. For example, it can remain in the brain for more than 20 years, while kidneys may retain mercury for 60 days.

Can mercury be the cause of infertility? Several studies have shown that mercury-containing compounds are effective spermicides. Mercury prevents sperm from picking up essential minerals, such as zinc, copper, iron, or manganese, needed for sperm to function. Mercury can also affect the ability of sperm to swim.

Is there any protection for the sperm? Selenium, a mineral that can bind to mercury and inactivate it, to the rescue! We know that selenium accumulates in the testes and is found in high amounts in ejaculate. The selenium is used up in the process of binding the mercury, so a good intake of selenium-containing foods (eggs, liver) or supplements in the diet may prove effective in combating the effects of mercury and other toxic metals.

There are also reports of women who worked in air polluted with mercury vapor, such as in dentistry or in factories that reclaim mercury. Almost 29% of the mercury-exposed women had hypermenorrhea—excessive bleeding from the uterus. Over 15% of these women experienced less than the normal amount of bleeding.

In another study of women working with fluorescent lamps containing mercury vapor, besides bleeding problems, there was a 46.7% incidence of anovulation (failure to ovulate or release an egg). In studies looking at female dentists, it was found that they had a higher rate of spontaneous abortions, especially with first pregnancies.

As harmful as mercury is to adults, it is even more harmful to the unborn child. To protect herself and her unborn child, a woman should **never** have mercury-containing fillings removed during pregnancy. The amount of mercury getting into the mother's bloodstream and to the baby could harm the unborn child. Mercury concentrations were measured in the body tissues of fetuses (obtained from medically necessary abortions) and in children (dying mainly from sudden infant death syndrome). The amount of mercury in the kidneys and liver of fetuses and in the kidney and cerebral cortex of the brain of infants correlated significantly with the number of dental amalgam fillings in the mother. The more fillings the mother had, the higher the level of mercury in the children's bodies! The study by Dr. G. Drasch published in the European Journal of Pediatrics in 1994, concluded that "unrestricted application of amalgam for dental restorations in women before and during their childbearing age should be reconsidered."

In 1987, the Swedish government health board declared publicly that amalgam was toxic and unsuitable as a dental filling material. As a first step, amalgam work in pregnant women was stopped, "in order to prevent damage to the fetus." Mercury can cross the placenta and cause birth defects. If fillings are to be removed, it should be done before pregnancy, or afterwards—but not during breast feeding because of the risk that the mercury can get into the milk.

Both Sides of the Fence

The American Dental Association (ADA) does not believe that dental mercury is a threat to humans. In a legal brief filed by their attorneys they said, "The ADA owes no legal duty of care to protect the public from allegedly dangerous products used by dentists."

What can a women do if she has a mouthful of mercury and is pregnant? This is where good nutrition and supplementation play a role. Antioxidant vitamins—vitamin C, vitamin E, beta-carotene, and others—can counteract the harmful effects of mercury on body tissues. We will talk more about key nutrients in chapter 2.

CHAPTER 2

The Right Diet for
Mothers-to-Be

Many people still believe that a baby can get all the nutrients it needs as it grows in the uterus from its mother's diet. While it's important to eat healthfully during pregnancy, it is even more important to eat the best diet possible *before* you get pregnant. This idea is called "receptive conception."

At the moment the sperm fertilizes the egg, everything your baby will need to grow and develop is in place. The key nutrients for dental health and growth of other body systems are available to the baby only if there are good stores of these nutrients in the body of the mother. The vitamins and minerals, proteins, and good fats have to be there before the new life begins. This is especially true when you remember that all the major organs—heart, brain, kidneys, and so on—are formed during the first few weeks of pregnancy. Many women don't realize they are pregnant until they miss their first menstrual period. By that time, major body systems have begun to form in the baby. If the nutrients are already there, your baby will get the best start in life. During pregnancy, additional nutrients must be obtained from the mother's diet or from supplements for the best growth and for good tooth development.

Some Key Nutrients for Prospective Mothers

Vitamin C

The principal function of vitamin C is to help make collagen, the main protein substance of the human body. Collagen is used to make all the connective tissue, cartilage, and tendons, including the tissue that anchors teeth in their sockets. Vitamin C is vital for wound repair, healthy gums, and the prevention of easy bruising. It plays a major role in immune system functioning, strengthening the immune cells such as the white blood cells that scavenge bacteria. In pregnant women, low vitamin C levels are found when there is premature rupture of fetal membranes ("my water broke"). The sac around the baby that contains the amniotic fluid (water) contains collagen for strength. A strong sac is less likely to rupture.

Several doctors report that daily doses of vitamin C resulted in shorter and less painful labor times, very few stretch marks, and no adverse reactions to the vitamin C in mother or baby. "The babies are healthy, pink, and squalling," said Robert S. Scott, M.D., former head of the Southern Women's Medical Group in Los Angeles, California, and a professor of obstetrics and gynecology at the University of Southern California. Vitamin C also reduces the risk of preeclampsia, a serious condition that may threaten the lives of both mother and child.

We recommend that vitamin C supplementation be started *before* conception if you have never taken it. It is not a good idea to suddenly start taking large doses, whether you are pregnant or not. Although up to 4000 mg (4 grams) of vitamin C has been given in the first three months of pregnancy, this level was reached by gradually increasing the amount over a period of several weeks. If you have been taking vitamin C, you can continue the amount, following these suggestions: To prevent stomach upset, always take vitamin C with food. Also, the form of vitamin C may make a difference. Ascorbic acid, which is another name for vitamin C, may cause problems such as gas and loose bowels in some people. Taking vitamin C in the form of calcium ascorbate (also called "buffered" or "nonacidic") may reduce or eliminate these problems.

Folic Acid

Women who do not have enough of the B vitamin folic acid at the time of conception and during pregnancy have a higher risk of having babies with birth defects, especially of the brain or spinal cord. Each year in the United States, about 4,000 pregnancies result in spina bifida (failure of the back bone to cover the spinal cord), or anencephaly (underdeveloped brain). The Public Health Service recommends that all women of childbearing age capable of becoming pregnant get 400 micrograms (mcg) of folic acid daily. The FDA now requires that all enriched cereal grains be fortified with folic acid.

To obtain the recommended amount (400 mcg before pregnancy and 800 mcg during pregnancy), women must either take a folic acid supplement daily or eat foods rich in folic acid. Such foods include green leafy vegetables like kale, spinach, beet greens, and chard. Other good sources are legumes (beans), asparagus, broccoli, cabbage, oranges, root vegetables, and whole grains.

Folic acid is important in preventing cleft lip and cleft lip/palate, which can cause abnormal growth of the teeth. These defects also cause feeding and speech problems and ear infections.

As reported in *Dentistry Today,* researchers believe that folic acid could prevent or decrease the risk of these birth defects. To test this belief, they studied 221 women planning to have a baby. Based on their genetic and medical histories, these women had a higher than normal risk for having a baby with a cleft palate. The women supplemented their diet with vitamins and high doses of folic acid taken three times daily beginning at least 2 months before they planned to conceive, and until at least the fourth month of pregnancy. The multivitamin supplement contained vitamins A (2,000 International Units, or IU), B_1 (1 mg), C (50 mg), D_3 (100 IU), B_5 (1 mg), E (2 mg), niacinamide (10 mg), and folic acid (10 mg) daily.

Researchers then compared the outcome of the women taking the supplements to women at risk of having a child with a cleft defect who did not take the supplements. Among the women who supplemented, only three mothers had infants born with cleft defect, a 65.4% decrease greater than was expected. The researchers concluded that a diet rich in vitamins and folic acid reduced the likelihood of an infant born with cleft palate in families at risk for this birth defect. The dosages of vitamins caused no side effects for the mothers participating in the study.

Another study on cleft defects and multivitamins found a 25% to 50% reduced risk of defects if the mother had used multivitamins containing folic acid during a period 1 month before and through 2 months after conception.

Vitamin B$_6$

Vitamin B$_6$ is important because of its role in reducing or eliminating the morning sickness that can make life miserable for a pregnant woman. Nausea and vomiting also deprive the unborn baby of needed nutrients. In studies, 30 mg a day of vitamin B$_6$ was found to significantly reduce the nausea of morning sickness.

"I'm a Believer" by Jean Barilla

When my daughter was pregnant with her first child, she started to suffer from morning sickness. I told her about vitamin B$_6$ and gave her 50 mg a day for a few days. The morning sickness disappeared. She then decided that it wasn't the B$_6$, and that the nausea had gone away on its own. She stopped the B$_6$. The morning sickness came back the next day. "Mom," she said, "give me the B$_6$. *Now* I believe it did the trick."

How to Prevent Morning Sickness: The best remedy for morning sickness is vitamin B$_6$ (see above).

If you want to use other methods, here are some that have been tried. They may work for you. You can try more than one suggestion. Remember, this is a condition that will gradually disappear.

- At night, place dry crackers, toast, or dry cereal beside your bed. Before you get out of bed in the morning, eat these foods slowly. Stay in bed for 15–20 minutes, then get up slowly and avoid unnecessary bending while dressing.
- Avoid rushing in the morning. Allow enough time for dressing, eating, morning chores, or getting to work.
- Chew foods well and eat slowly. Keep portion sizes small.

Choose foods you really enjoy and have a pleasant atmosphere when you eat.

- Certain smells may bother you, such as those from cooking, frying, or brewing coffee. Try to keep pots covered; use the oven.
- Eat only solid foods early in the day. Divide breakfast into two or three small snacks and eat at 1-hour intervals. Use cooked fruit or well-ripened bananas, no juices. No fried or fatty foods. Later on, sip liquids if thirsty: clear tea or coffee (decaffeinated) or skim milk.
- Fat, oil, and mayonnaise may cause nausea. Trim fat from meat before cooking. Use very little salad dressing; control the amount of butter added to cooked foods. Use jam, fruit spreads, jelly, honey, or molasses on toast or bread instead of butter. Bake, broil, roast, simmer, or stew meats. Avoid fried foods. Use no gravy or cream sauces.
- Keep busy. Get out to walk, visit friends and relatives. Just being out in the fresh air may help.
- Avoid taking prenatal vitamins and iron when nauseated. You should always take vitamins and minerals with food, as they absorb better.
- In a recent study, ginger provided significant relief for many of the 30 pregnant women in a study of morning sickness. It has been used safely for over 2,500 years for stomach and intestinal problems.

Calcium

Calcium is important for building strong bones and healthy teeth. But it has many other functions in the body. Calcium is needed to regulate the heartbeat, ensure normal clotting of blood, aid the contraction of muscles, and produce enzyme activity. Low calcium contributes to high blood pressure, osteoporosis, and colon cancer. In pregnancy, calcium may prevent the development of *hypertension* (high blood pressure) and *preeclampsia* (a serious condition associated with elevated blood pressure, fluid retention, and protein loss in the urine).

The main source of calcium is dairy products. Vegetables can also be a good source of calcium and are especially good for women who have lactose (milk sugar) intolerance or allergies to dairy foods. Carrots are high in calcium.

Not all vegetables with significant amounts of calcium are good sources of calcium in the diet; some contain oxalic acid, a naturally occurring substance that makes the calcium unavailable to the body. Beet greens, Swiss chard, and spinach have such a high content of oxalic acid that they are a poor source of calcium. Other greens, such as turnip, mustard, collard, kale, and broccoli, have little oxalic acid and so the calcium they contain is available to the body. Kale is actually higher in calcium than milk and the calcium is very absorbable. Remember, though, it takes about 11/2 cups of most of these vegetables to equal the amount of calcium in a glass of milk.

Magnesium

In many women who have leg cramps during pregnancy, researchers have found that magnesium levels were lower in these women compared with women who didn't have leg cramps. The recommended dietary allowance of magnesium is 450 mg. The average amount pregnant women get from their diets is 35 to 58% of this amount. Even prenatal supplements seldom have more than 100 mg. Leg cramps can also be helped with vitamin B_1 and vitamin B_6, both found to be lower in pregnant women.

Zinc

The critical need for zinc during pregnancy is finally being realized based on studies acceptable to the medical community. Zinc is needed to make the proteins that will become the baby's muscles, and that will be used to make enzymes and proteins—it is even needed to make the baby's DNA, or genetic material. A low zinc intake may therefore affect the growth and development of the baby.

A study done at the University of Glasgow and at the University of Birmingham in England measured zinc levels in the placenta and umbilical cord in mothers who had given birth to normal-weight or low-birth-weight infants. A larger placenta was associated with a higher infant birth weight. Although the zinc concentrations in the placenta were similar in both groups, the zinc in the umbilical cord blood of mothers with normal-weight babies was significantly higher than in mothers of low-birth-weight infants. These mothers had enough zinc to reach their babies. The researchers concluded that lower zinc concentrations in umbilical cord blood might retard growth of infants. Another study was done at the University of Alabama at Birmingham. Five hundred healthy pregnant women with below-normal blood levels of zinc took part in the study. All of the infants born to women taking 25 mg of supplemental zinc a day had greater birth weights and larger head circumferences than babies born to women not receiving the zinc.

Zinc is found in many foods, but levels are highest in seafood, meat, nuts, and milk.

Vitamin A and Birth Defects

Every pregnant woman should know that too much Vitamin A in certain forms may be harmful to the baby, causing birth defects. Women should not take synthetic vitamin A supplements (of over 10,000 IU) but should get naturally occurring vitamin A from whole foods or as beta carotene supplements.

We know that vitamin A is essential for normal fetal growth and development and that a deficiency of vitamin A has also been linked to birth defects. So what is the final word? A study conducted by National Institutes of Health researchers tried to determine whether there were risks associated with taking vitamin A during pregnancy. The researchers looked at vitamin A intake in 935 women whose children had neural tube defects, had other birth defects, or were healthy. The women were asked how much vitamin A they ate from dietary supplements, fortified cold cereals, and other food sources (such as organ meats). They compared the various levels of vitamin A intake to whether or not the woman's child had a birth defect.

They found "no significant increase" in birth defects with vitamin A doses of over 8,000 IU up to 10,000 IU, either as supplements alone or as supplements and fortified foods. . . . These findings support the claim that moderate doses of vitamin A are not teratogenic [birth-defect-causing]. The researchers do caution that moderate amounts of vitamin A are safe during pregnancy, but that high amounts should be avoided.

We recommend that you take no more than 10,000 IU of vitamin A from a supplement. Pregnant women can take part or all of their vitamin A as beta-carotene, which the body can convert into vitamin A. Take at least 5,000 IU as vitamin A and 5,000 IU or more as beta-carotene. Beta-carotene can be taken as a supplement if enough of the foods that contain it are not eaten.

You will need to eat a lot of vegetables and fruits to get enough vitamin A, since it takes 6 units (IU) of beta-carotene to produce 1 unit of vitamin A. With low-fat diets, bile (a body chemical that helps digest fats) is not released in the intestine. Bile is needed to convert beta-carotene and other carotenes from vegetables into vitamin A. So if your diet is low-fat you may not make much vitamin A from beta-carotene. Foods that contain vitamin A (already formed) include liver, egg yolks, cod liver oil, and butterfat (butter and cream). Some of these foods should be part of your diet so that you can get natural vitamin A and be able to convert more beta-carotene into vitamin A as your body needs it.

Multivitamins

Evidence shows that multivitamin/mineral supplements (containing folic acid) will prevent several types of birth defects. A large study of 1,430 pregnant women found that those women who took multivitamin/mineral supplements during the first and second trimester had a twofold reduction in the risk of premature delivery. The risk of having a very premature delivery (less than 33 weeks gestation) was reduced more than four times for women who took the vitamins starting in the first trimester, while those who started in the second trimester had a twofold reduction.

Heart defects can also be prevented by multivitamin supplementation. A study conducted by researchers at the Division of Birth Defects and Developmental Disabilities at the Centers for Disease Control and Prevention looked at infants having major heart defects. They found that the risk of heart defects was decreased by 64% in infants of women who took multivitamins regularly from 3 months before conception through the third month.

According to the American Dental Association, the best thing an expectant mother can do for her baby's teeth is to follow the rules for her own dental health:

- Eat a balanced diet containing protein, carbohydrates, fats, and water
- Brush and floss daily to remove plaque
- Avoid sweet or starchy snacks
- Have regular dental examinations

Protein

Protein and its components (amino acids) are important for growth and repair of the body. Of the 22 amino acids that make up protein, at least 8 are essential. This means they must be taken in the form of food or food supplements at the same time and each day.

During pregnancy many things grow: the placenta, the baby, and structures in the mother's body such as milk glands. Such growth requires a good protein intake. Proteins are also needed to make enzymes that help get oxygen and nutrients through the blood for mother and child.

Proteins help create hair, skin, muscle, and connective tissue and help maintain water balance in the cells of the body. Other proteins are needed to form blood, immune-system-enhancing antibodies, brain transmitters, and all the hormones of the body. Protein is also necessary for all the repair mechanisms in the body—for healing tissues and repairing the DNA, the genetic material itself.

Protein deficiency can create abnormalities in growth and tissue development as well as physical and mental impairment. Given these many roles, it is important for pregnant women to eat adequate amounts of protein. It is also important to eat protein that is usable by the body.

Proteins are rated in terms of their Net Protein Utilization (NPU) value. The egg is generally considered to be the most usable protein source and is thus used as a basis for comparing other proteins. Proteins derived from animal products are high in usable protein and generally contain all the essential amino acids. Plant proteins can also supply sufficient protein, yet more often require eating a greater amount and combining vegetable sources to ensure that necessary essential amino acids are consumed.

For example, combining rice and beans, or pasta (or bread) and beans, will result in the right amounts of essential amino acids being eaten. Raw living foods, such as yogurt and buttermilk, along with sprouted-grain breads and sprouted grains and beans, also supply sufficiently high amounts of protein.

The government's Recommended Daily Allowance (RDA) for protein is 0.36 grams per pound of body weight for an adult. This works out to 45 grams per day for a 120-pound woman and 54 grams per day for a 150-pound man. Many nutritionists feel that these amounts should be about 10 grams per day higher for optimal health. Pregnant women require an extra 30 grams of protein and nursing mothers an extra 20 grams in addition to normal levels.

When you eat the required amount of protein is very important. We should have at least one third of the total requirement for the day at breakfast. For a 120-pound pregnant woman, that would be about 20 to 25 grams.

A typical American breakfast of cereal, toast, and coffee supplies only 2 to 4 grams of protein. Following is a list of foods that contain protein. The * in front of some of the foods means that the protein is incomplete (doesn't contain all 8 essential amino acids) or of low quality. These proteins must be combined with some animal protein, or a larger amount of a complementary vegetable protein, in order to be as useful to the body as a similar amount of animal protein.

The best sources of complete protein are meat, fish, cheese, and eggs. Foods such as breads, potatoes, cold cereals, and pancakes have very little protein. Other vegetables, such as green beans, spinach, carrots, broccoli, and beets (not listed) have only 1 to 3 grams of protein in a moderate serving, and the protein is of low quality. Of course these vegetables are good sources of other needed nutrients such as vitamins and minerals. There are no fruits on the list since they have even less protein than vegetables.

SOURCES OF PROTEIN

Food	grams of protein
Chicken, 3 ounces	23
Fish, 3 ounces	23
Steak, hamburger, 3 ounces	22
Cheese (cheddar, Swiss), 2 ounces	17
* Baked beans, lentils, 1 cup	15
Cottage cheese, ½ cup	14
* Peanut butter, 3 tablespoons	13
* Tofu, 1 cake 2 ¾" x ½" x 1"	9
* Soy grits, 2 tablespoons	9
Milk, 8 ounces	8
Yogurt, 1 cup	8
* Wheat germ, ¼ cup	8
* Almonds, ¼ cup	6
* Oatmeal, 1 cup	5
* Brewer's yeast, one tablespoon	4
Bacon, 2 slices	4
Cream cheese, 2 ounces	2
* Rice, 1 cup	4
* Cold cereal, 1 ounce	2
* Bread, 1 slice	2
Pancake, 1"–4"	2
* Potato, 1 medium	2

*Incomplete or low-quality

Carbohydrates

There are two types of carbohydrates: complex and simple. The complex carbohydrates include vegetables, fruits, grain products (cereals, pasta), and rice. Simple carbohydrates are what we think of as sugar: refined white sugar, syrups, jams and jellies, honey, and so on.

Sugar

Women are consuming more sugar than ever before, and there is evidence that it can affect their pregnancies. A study at the University of Medicine and Dentistry of New Jersey compared pregnant women with high-sugar diets with those who limited their sugar intakes. The women on the high-sugar diets were twice as likely to deliver small-for-gestational-age infants. The babies were not premature, but they were smaller than full-term babies should be. Although recommendations for sugar are around 10% of total calories, the women in the study consumed sugar at upwards of 44% of total calories.

Foods high in carbohydrates, primarily sugars (sweets such as cakes, cookies, dried fruits, and caramels) are easily fermented and combine with plaque, the sticky layer of harmful bacteria found in the mouth. This combination results in the production of acid that is capable of dissolving the mineral components of the enamel and dentin of the teeth.

Each time you eat sugary foods, acid attacks the tooth enamel and continues to attack it for at least 20 minutes. Brushing your teeth after a sweet snack will help, but you can't count on it to save your teeth from the effects of a high-carbohydrate, high-sugar diet. Plaque under the gum where the toothbrush can't reach can continue the acid production.

This kind of diet has an effect on the metabolism within the tooth that makes it more susceptible to decay.

Fats: Good Fats Make a Difference

Although pregnancy is not the time to be worrying about losing weight, it is the time to be choosy about the fats that you eat. There are good fats and bad fats. The message to take home is that you can cut down on fats if you cut down on the bad fats, but you don't want to cut down on the good ones.

Docosahexaenoic acid (DHA) is one of the good fats. It belongs to the omega-3 group of fats and is found in human breast milk, seafood and fish oil, and eggs. This is the primary structural fat, essential to infant brain and eye development. It is so essential that if a mother and infant are deficient, the child's nervous system may never fully develop, causing a lifetime of unexplained emotional, learning, and immune system disorders.

Referring to omega-3 fats, researchers from the Mayo Clinic

suggest that "this important fat be supplemented in every pregnancy, and that refined and hydrogenated fats be avoided during this critical period." Hydrogenated fats, as you will learn later, are even more harmful than cholesterol.

Fetuses depend primarily upon their mothers' stores of DHA, which they receive through the placenta. While adults can make a limited amount of DHA from certain vegetable oils, a baby's body cannot make DHA fast enough to meet the needs of its rapidly developing brain. While you are pregnant you can supply an adequate amount to your baby by eating lots of DHA-rich foods or by taking DHA supplements throughout pregnancy. Foods such as eggs, salmon, tuna, and sardines contain ample amounts of DHA. Breast milk will be your infant's only source of DHA. Unfortunately, American mothers typically have low breast milk DHA levels. Formula-fed infants in the United States are deprived of DHA because most American infant formulas do not contain DHA. A debate still rages on, however, as to whether DHA is necessary in formula.

Fear of Eating Fat (From the *Mittelman's Holistic Dental Digest Plus*)

Fear of eating fat distorts food choices. Many people forsake nutritious foods with moderate amounts of fat while eating unnutritious foods just because they are "low-fat."

For example, some people avoid cheese and lean red meat but regularly eat cake, pie, or other desserts that actually contain more fat. People substitute low-protein complex carbohydrates such as white rice, pasta, and cold cereals with a fraction of the nutrients in highly nutritious lean meat, poultry, fish, nuts, and beans. Refined white flour products such as white bread and pasta, white rice, and cold cereals should not be put in the same category as 100% whole-grain breads and cereals, beans, and root vegetables.

Possibly worse, people believe that low-fat, high-sugar desserts and flavored yogurt are all right just because they're low in fat.

Here are some comparisons of fat content (in grams per serving):

Apple pie	16 g	Lean broiled steak, 4 oz raw	5 g
Danish pastry	14 g	Cheese, 1 oz	7–9 g

Chocolate cake	12 g	Cottage cheese (1/2 cup)	5 g
Bologna, 3 oz	24 g	Chicken without skin	3–6 g
French fries	12–18 g	Milk, 2% fat, 1 cup	5 g
Chocolate candy bar	13–18 g	Salmon, canned, 3.5 oz	6 g

Water

Most people don't think of water as a nutrient. It may surprise you to learn that water is the most important substance you can put into your body!

The detoxification and waste-removal systems of your body, especially the kidneys, need water to do their jobs. When cells don't have enough water, they can't make hormones, convert nutrients to energy, or excrete waste products. Cells that are dehydrated (low on water) are smaller and function poorly.

Especially during pregnancy, water is important because the mother will have to detoxify not only her own wastes, but also those of her baby. Since she will need to drink eight glasses a day or more of water, it would be wise to use bottled or filtered water.

Natural Wisdom

Do women ever eat properly (with no counseling) when pregnant? One study looked at the dietary behavior of a group of women in early pregnancy and a group of nonpregnant women. The study found that pregnant women do eat differently from nonpregnant women.

Intake of zinc and vitamin C, protein and sodium were higher and alcohol lower in the pregnant women. The group of pregnant women also tended to eat more milk and fruit and less chocolate, cakes, and pastries compared to nonpregnant women. These differences were not due to the specific knowledge about nutrition that the pregnant women had, but just the choice by pregnant women to eat healthier. Both the pregnant and the nonpregnant women had the same nutrition knowledge.

The Brewer Diet for Pregnancy

In 1983, Gail Sforza Brewer and her husband Thomas H. Brewer, M.D., wrote the now classic book *The Brewer Medical Diet for Normal and High-Risk Pregnancy.* We believe that the diet they recommended (with some modifications based on current knowledge) is still one of the best diets for pregnant women. The Brewer Medical Diet for Pregnancy was developed with over 30 years of research and clinical work with pregnant women.

The Brewers make the statement that "every pregnant woman we see is malnourished until proved otherwise—and the proof doesn't come until after the baby is born, and maybe not until after the child has entered school." Hundreds of improvements in the health of both mother and baby come from better nutrition, and the Brewers give many examples. A pediatrician (who you would think should know better) developed toxemia and had a 4-pound baby after following a low-calorie, low-salt diet. *Toxemia of pregnancy* refers to metabolic disturbances and is also called *preeclampsia.* She then had a full-term, full-sized baby with no toxemia the second time when she salted to taste and ate good foods to appetite. One woman ate well but not enough and delivered a 2-pound baby who died 10 days later. With her next pregnancy she doubled her food intake and delivered a healthy 7-pound baby. Another woman with severe high blood pressure lost four babies on her regular antihypertension regimen of reduced salt, diuretics, and tranquilizers while pregnant. At age 40, she delivered a healthy 6-pound, 6-ounce baby after resuming salt intake and eliminating drugs. Her blood pressure came down during pregnancy, even though she was under enormous emotional and physical stress.

Good nutrition promotes an increase in the mother's blood supply. Extra blood is needed for nutrients from the mother to get across the placenta to the baby. The Brewers' general recommendations are designed to ensure that the baby gets a steady supply of nutrition: don't go more than 12 hours without food; eat breakfast, a midmorning snack, lunch, a midafternoon snack, and a snack before bed. They even suggest that you can eat at least once during the night if you wake up hungry. The following diet covers all the basic nutrition groups needed for your health and that of your developing baby.

Group 1: milk, milk products, calcium-fortified milk substitutes (soy), four glasses of milk or its equivalent, such as 1 cup of yogurt for a cup of milk.

Group 2: calcium replacements (supplements) as needed—when drinking soy milk, or carrying twins, or when you can't drink all the milk recommended. The RDA for calcium for a pregnant woman is 1,200 mg a day.

Group 3: eggs, two a day.

Group 4: meats, seafood, and meat substitutes (cheese, beans, nuts, seeds, and pasta), two servings. For those women who don't eat meat or fish, alternative combinations include:

Rice with beans, cheese, sesame seeds, or milk
Cornmeal with beans, cheese, tofu, or milk
Beans with rice, bulgur, cornmeal, wheat noodles, sesame seeds, or milk
Peanuts with sunflower seeds, or milk
Whole-wheat bread or noodles with beans, cheese, peanut butter, milk, or tofu

For each serving of meat, you can substitute these amounts of cheese:

Cottage: 6 oz	Brick: 4 oz
Swiss: 3 oz	Camembert: 6 oz
Cheddar: 3 oz	Monterey Jack: 4 oz
Muenster: 4 oz	Longhorn: 3 oz

Group 5: fresh dark-green and leafy veggies: kale, spinach, mustard, beet, collard, dandelion, or turnip greens, broccoli, two servings.

Group 6: whole grains (whole oats, whole-wheat bread, rolls, cereal, pancakes; whole corn and products made from spelt and kamut), whole-grain rice, starchy veggies (peas, lima beans), fruits (banana), five servings.

Group 7: vitamin C–rich foods: citrus fruits (orange, grapefruit), green peppers, strawberries, tomatoes, mangos, papaya, whole potato, cabbage, Brussels sprouts, broccoli. Two servings.

Group 8: good fats and oils: olive oil, canola oil, fish oils (from oily fish such as mackerel, sardines), flaxseed oil, nuts, butter (if organic), five servings.

Group 9: vitamin A–rich foods (cantaloupe, apricots, sweet potatoes, carrots), one serving.

Group 10: liver, once per week. Liver should be organic. An alternative is to take liver capsules made from the liver of animals not fed hormones and antibiotics.

Group 11: salt and sodium sources (soy sauce, kelp, sea salt), unlimited.

Group 12: water, unlimited.

Group 13: healthy snacks, unlimited.

Group 14: optional supplements: If you follow the diet to the letter, you probably won't need more than a good prenatal multivitamin containing 800 mcg of folic acid. But you do need extra supplements if you bruise easily or if gums bleed (increase vitamin C to 1 or 2 grams (1,000 mg to 2,000 mg) a day. Increase gradually, by 500 mg at a time over a period of 2 weeks. If acidic vitamin C (ascorbic acid) produces digestive upsets, try the buffered vitamin C (calcium ascorbate). If there is recent weight loss before conception, or if you were taking birth control pills and not adding extra B vitamins, especially folic acid, to your diet, you need extra vitamins and minerals. Also in the case of twins, stress, if you are a vegetarian or sick, you will need extra supplements.

NOTE: The authors of this book don't agree that supplements should be "optional." Since the Brewers wrote their book, the burden of toxic chemicals and food additives and food adulterations has increased substantially. We want to stress that supplements are important for optimal nutrition for mother and baby. Even with the rare mother who will stick to the diet to the letter, our foods are not as nutrient-dense and chemical-free as those of our ancestors. It's almost impossible to be perfect—to eat right 100% of the time, avoid chemicals and pollutants, and so on. So everyone is under stress from the environment, and just getting nutrients from the average diet is not enough for good health.

The Brewers on protein: below 75 grams a day of high-quality, complete protein, the rates of serious pregnancy complications rise proportionately. Vitamin E, 200–400 mg per day can alleviate many problems with varicosities of the legs, vulva, and anus (hemorrhoids) without any harmful effects on the pregnancy. Brewer recommends a diet of 3,000 calories per day. Why? For fuel—so you won't start using up the protein you eat. Without the calories, your body burns some protein, leaving less for growth and maintenance of body tissues—your and the baby's body and brain, and so on. Especially for women who are working full time or doing vigorous sports programs, or looking after three or four other children, calorie needs are high. Most diets given in doctor's offices don't consider activity levels.

If you are not obese and your calories are one-third less than what you need, then half the protein you eat is going to be burned for energy. If you are eating 90 grams of protein this leaves 45, far below the 75 grams needed for a nutritionally secure pregnancy. "Eat to appetite, nutritious foods from the diet list," say the Brewers—not junk food.

Weight: If a woman is underweight, the first 20 pounds may only bring her to what she should have weighed to start with. Then she may gain another 20 to 40 pounds, the pregnancy gain. The number of pounds on the scale is absolutely irrelevant to the outcome of pregnancy, say the Brewers. Nobody can tell, just from weighing, whether the weight gained represents additional fat, muscle, water, or baby. What matters is the adequacy of the mother's nutrition. According to Dr. Brewer, "The food you eat every day while you are pregnant builds the bones, muscle and brain of your baby. Pounds gained while you are on a good diet protect and prepare you for labor and breast-feeding. If you gain a few extra pounds during this pregnancy from eating a nutritious, balanced diet, it won't hurt you or the baby—even if you gain fifty or sixty pounds. Worry if you don't gain enough."

When Jean Barilla's daughter was pregnant with her first child, she gained almost 50 pounds, eating a healthy diet and taking vitamin and mineral supplements. The baby was born (5 pounds, 7 ounces) healthy and strong—she could turn herself over at 4 days of age! The author's daughter went back to her usual 128 pounds before she finished nursing.

Salt: "Salt to taste." According to Dr. Brewer, you need more sodium (salt) because it helps keep the placenta adequately supplied with blood, so it can pump nutrients to the developing baby. Your body signals when it needs more sodium by the taste buds on your tongue and in your cheeks that are sensitive to salt. When you need more, your food tastes flat and unappetizing, and so you add some salt (preferably sea salt, which contains minerals). This doesn't mean you coat everything with salt. If your heart and kidneys are healthy and you take in enough fluids, salt will not hurt you. If levels of salt do get too high, the kidney excretes the excess into the urine. Having enough potassium in the diet (bananas, oranges) will prevent salt levels from getting too high.

During pregnancy you need sodium to keep the correct concentration of salt in the blood. The salt helps hold the extra fluid for the expanded blood volume needed for the baby; keeps the correct concentration of salt in the amniotic fluid that surrounds the baby (and that the baby drinks); aids your heart, which needs to do extra work pumping the extra blood around; and helps leg muscles, which may cramp with low sodium.

The swelling of the body that accompanies a normal pregnancy is due to placental hormones, like those that make you swell just before your period. The amount of these hormones increases; by the eighth month, in the well-nourished mother, the placenta makes, every day, the equivalent of the hormones in a hundred birth control pills. This swelling is not hazardous to you or your baby. It's a natural way for your body to prepare for labor and breast feeding by storing fluids you may need to avoid dehydration if your labor lasts a long time and to establish and maintain quality milk production.

On a good diet, your liver makes enough albumin, a protein that holds the water in your blood vessels where it belongs. Ten to 15 pounds of water can be held. On a poor diet, the water leaks out of the vessels because of low levels of albumin. The water goes into your tissues. This is the swelling that causes trouble. Blood volume drops and the placenta is not properly perfused (filled) with blood, and nutrients and oxygen have difficulty getting to your baby.

If this continues, other critical body organs, like the kidneys, liver, heart, lungs, and brain, become adversely affected by the dwindling blood supply. The kidneys respond, for example, by raising blood pressure, and the baby begins to suffer intrauterine malnutrition. This is diagnosed after a few weeks when the baby's failure to grow is noted; it is called intrauterine growth retardation. If caught early enough, it can be reversed with nutritional intervention.

Good nutrition makes labor easier: collagen (connective tissue) is laid down in large quantities by well-fed women during pregnancy. Collagen gives strength and elasticity to the tissues that have to stretch during pregnancy. It requires protein, vitamin C, vitamin A, zinc, and the amino acid lysine to make good connective tissue. Even though the baby of a well-nourished woman may be larger, the uterus (with its healthy connective tissue) is strong enough to deliver it. Also, a well-fed mother's placenta will make a lot of hormones that relax the pelvic ligaments so it will "give" more during labor. Episiotomies may not be necessary if the skin is stretchy and doesn't tear easily as with poorly nourished women. The placenta is anchored to the wall of the uterus by collagen strands that are stronger when you are well nourished. This helps prevent abruption of the placenta (premature separation), which can be fatal to mother and baby.

What to Avoid During Pregnancy (Drugs, Toxins)

There are many *teratogenic agents* (those that can cause birth defects), including drugs, environmental chemicals and toxins, and infections. Some of these can cause major defects if the fetus is exposed during a critical period in development, but may cause no harm at other times. The first 13 weeks of pregnancy are the time when all major organs are forming in the fetus. Insults to the body at this time will cause abnormal development (shape) of these organs. After this time effects may be limited to growth retardation in organs or body size and defects in the function of the organs. Not all babies will be affected in the same way after exposure to a toxic substance. There is individual variation from one person to another in susceptibility to a dose of a known teratogenic agent. Because of differences in genetics, for example, each child of a chronic alcoholic may display different features of fetal alcohol syndrome. Before you take *any* medication, including nonprescription (over-the-counter) medications and herbs, discuss it with your doctor or other health care professional.

The U.S. Food and Drug Administration (FDA) has classified drugs (and nutrients) into five categories of risk (A, B, C, D, and X) for use during pregnancy. Your physician will be aware of these classifications if he or she must prescribe a drug. You can check the status of the drug (or other substance) as well before you take it.

For the following substances (not a complete list), there is strong evidence that they cause birth defects:

Alcohol: nutritional deficiency, smoking, and multiple drug use make it difficult to interpret the results of alcohol, but fetuses of women who ingest six drinks per day have a 40% risk of developing features of fetal alcohol syndrome. Researchers are not really sure about the risk due to one or two drinks per day, but this amount may cause a small reduction in average birth weight. Is it worth the risk of having a smaller-than-normal baby?

Cocaine: abnormalities of the heart, limbs, face, and genitourinary tract; microcephaly (tiny head); growth restriction; strokes.

Lead: increased abortion rate, stillbirths, brain abnormalities.

Lithium: given for manic depression; causes congenital heart disease for first trimester exposure; in last month of pregnancy may produce toxic effects on the thyroid, kidneys, and neuromuscular systems.

Tetracycline: an antibiotic often given for acne or lung infection; causes hypoplasia (undergrowth) of tooth enamel; the antibiotic incorporates right into bone and teeth weakening them, and may produce ugly, yellow-brown discoloration of permanent teeth if the drug is given from 18 weeks before birth to 10 months after birth.

Valproic acid: given for seizures; causes neural tube defects, especially spina bifida, minor facial defects.

Cytomegalovirus infection: severe disorders and damage of the brain and eyes, mental retardation, hearing loss.

Rubella infection: microcephaly, mental retardation, cataracts, deafness, congenital heart disease; all organs may be affected.

Syphilis infection: if severe, the fetus dies; if mild, detectable abnormalities of skin, teeth, and bones.

Radiation: microcephaly, mental retardation.

Other substances not documented as teratogens but with some evidence of causing birth defects:

Acetaminophen	Hair spray
Acyclovir	Marijuana
Antihistamines	Minor tranquilizers
Aspartame	Oral contraceptives
Aspirin	Occupational chemical agents
Caffeine	Pesticides
Vaginal spermicides	Trimethoprim-sulfamethoxazole (antibiotic)

Herpes Simplex Type 2 virus Parvovirus B_{19}
Electromagnetic fields from video display terminals
Heat

SOURCE: *American College of Obstetrics and Gynecology Educational Bulletin,* Number 236, April 1997.

Coffee and the Unborn Baby

Can coffee affect the unborn baby? In a study of 356 mother/baby pairs who had intrauterine growth retardation, it was found that 85.4% of the mothers whose babies had this growth deficiency drank coffee compared to 70.5% of mothers who didn't drink coffee and who had babies that were of normal size at birth. Although an increased risk is reported for women who drank at least 300 mg of cafeinated coffee daily (equivalent to about 3 cups), in this study the risk of smaller babies was significant even for women who drank less than 1 cup of coffee daily. Caffeine can also interfere with sleep by making mother and baby jittery. It's also a diuretic and will cause frequent urination, also disrupting sleep.

CHAPTER 3

Breast Feeding: A Vital Role in Prevention

What is the most important thing to do after a baby is born to avoid dental problems later? Make sure the child has regular dental checkups? Use the right toothpaste? Avoid sugar?

This may be the usual advice, but we would say something else. The most important thing is to make sure the baby is breast-fed. The human race has survived on human milk for 4 million years. It is the most nutritionally perfect food available for human babies.

Why Breast-Feed?

There are many reasons to breast-feed your child. First of all, breast milk protects against infection. Second, it contains growth regulators specifically for the newborn. Third, human milk contains the lowest amount of protein of any mammal milk. This is actually desirable, because babies don't need strong muscles so early. In fact, formula-fed babies are often heavier than breast-fed ones because of the higher protein content of commercial milk. Starting out heavy in life is not a good thing; it can result in problems later on, as you will see.

What babies need most is the right type of nutrition for their large and rapidly growing brains. Brain cells keep growing from birth until a baby is at least 6 months old. For the best possible brain growth, human infants need milk high in lactose (milk sugar) and essential fatty acids, such as DHA—and that is what breast milk gives them.

Breast milk also has the right *types* of protein for your baby. The amino acid *taurine,* found in the protein of breast milk, protects nerve cells and helps them grow properly. Breast milk contains high amounts of taurine, while cow's milk and prepared formulas contain almost no taurine. Human infants can't make taurine in their bodies (as adults can), and therefore need a regular dietary supply. Taurine helps the cells in the brain and eye by protecting them against toxins or oxidants (chemicals that damage cells). A study of premature infants fed mother's milk early in life found that these infants had significantly higher intelligence quotients (IQs) at 7 ½ to 8 years of age than those who were bottle-fed.

Some amino acids (the building blocks of proteins), such as phenylalanine and tyrosine, are present in low concentrations in human milk. This is good because the infant's liver is slow to develop the ability to use these amino acids, and high levels may strain their delicate systems. On the other hand, infant formula contains proteins that are changed during the manufacturing process and are not as nourishing for your baby. Cow's milk also contains many amino acids that cause allergic reactions in infants.

Newborns' stomachs are immature and have low levels of acid and the enzyme *pepsin,* which are needed to digest foods. Although pepsin helps digest proteins, this lack of pepsin is good for breast-fed infants because some important proteins in breast milk should not be broken down or digested. These proteins, which come from the mother, are called *immunoglobulins* and are part of her immune system. They can survive passage through the baby's stomach and can get to the intestines where they defend against infectious organisms.

Therefore, although babies are born with low levels of immunoglobulins, they receive them from the mother when they are breast-fed. Otherwise, they do not get this protection.

Babies fed cow's milk are at a disadvantage because cow's milk contains too much protein for human babies. As a result, the baby's intestine collects undigested protein, which gets into the baby's bloodstream to cause food hypersensitivity (allergies).

The differences in the proteins cause the formula-fed infant to have higher levels of insulin that may affect blood sugar (see below).

The widespread feeding of infants with cow's milk and formula has risen over the past 60 years. Although infant formulas based on cow's milk have been changed by adding some of the missing components that are known, often the amounts are far from the values found in breast milk. Some key nutrients are missing altogether. The fat content of breast milk is almost impossible to duplicate. There may be over 400 different types of fat in the milk of each species. Human breast milk contains fats that are easily absorbed by human infants. This is important because the fat tends to bring with it some of the calcium and fat-soluble vitamins. The fats also give breast-fed babies a sweeter smell than that of cow's-milk-fed babies.

Breast milk is also high in cholesterol—in this case a good thing. Because of the high level of cholesterol in breast milk, the baby's body doesn't make cholesterol—an ability that will be retained in later life. Formula-fed infants, on the other hand, have lower cholesterol levels, so they make cholesterol. They will not have the same protection as a breast-fed infant.

Breast milk contains enzymes that break down and digest fats. Lower amounts of fat is found in the stool of infants fed mother's milk compared to those on formula. This means that the baby has absorbed good unsaturated fat (palmitic, stearic, oleic, and linoleic) that the baby needs. Cow's milk contains saturated fats that are not as good for your baby as unsaturated fats.

Do breast-fed infants need vitamin supplements? Some researchers think that breast fed infants need iron. However, although the amount of iron in breast milk is very low (0.3 milligrams of iron per liter of milk), the infant absorbs almost half of it. In contrast, while iron-fortified formulas contain 10 to 20 milligrams of iron per liter, babies absorb only 4% of that iron. Not getting enough vitamin D can cause *rickets,* a disease that results in softening and bending of the bones. Although the amounts of vitamin D in breast milk are small, rickets is uncommon in the breast-fed baby. This may be because, like iron, the vitamin D in breast milk is easily absorbed by the baby.

There are also substances in breast milk that help with absorption of vitamin D. Vitamin D supplementation may be necessary if a mother and her baby cannot get enough sunlight—such as in the winter. When the sun shines on exposed skin, vitamin D is made in the skin. However, Baby needs only a few minutes of sun exposure a day. Commercial infant formulas usually contain 300 to 400 International Units (IU) of vitamin D. This amount is recommended for breast-fed babies deprived of sunlight and may be enough to prevent rickets. The mother who breast-feeds her baby may want to take vitamin D supplements (400 IU) or drink milk with that amount to provide the best conditions for her baby's growth.

How Breast Feeding Helps Your Baby

Colostrum (early milk) and breast milk contain white blood cells that absorb harmful materials so that the body can get rid of them. These cells help prevent infections and viruses. Breast milk also contains a friendly bacterium, *Lactobacillus bifidus,* which prevents overgrowth of harmful bacteria in the infant's intestines. Breast-fed babies have fewer hospitalizations for infectious diseases and fewer episodes of otitis media (ear infections), respiratory infections, meningitis, and bacteremias.

Breast milk may even have a protective effect against cancer. A study compared 201 children with cancer between the ages of 1.5 and 15 years and 181 children without cancer. Children breast-fed for more than 6 months were significantly less likely to have cancer than those breast-fed for lesser periods or who were formula-fed. The fad of not breast-feeding infants during the 1950s and 1960s may be partially responsible for today's higher rates of cancer and other immunological disorders in adults.

Breast feeding can also reduce the risk of developing juvenile diabetes. Breast-fed babies also have less frequent episodes of food allergies, eczema, rhinitis, and asthma.

Feeding cow's milk to human infants may turn them into baby cows—at least as far as their stomachs are concerned. Cows have a stomach with four compartments, with one used for fermenting food. Bacteria in the cow's stomach do the fermenting. Much of the colic that babies frequently get after drinking cow's milk is due to fermentation by the same bacteria found in the cow's stomach. Humans don't normally have this type of fermenting bacteria, as human milk discourages the growth of bacteria that produce toxic products leading to indigestion. The unique nutrients in breast milk may even help the baby's stomach and intestines to develop properly. The American Academy of Pediatrics strongly recommends that full-term infants be breast-fed exclusively for at least 1 year.

Here are some more ways breast milk makes your baby healthier:

- Formula feeding increases a baby girl's risk of developing breast cancer in later life. Women who were breast-fed as children, even if only for a short time, had a 25% lower risk of developing breast cancer than women who were bottle-fed as infants.
- Breast milk helps pass meconium, the sticky tarlike substance babies have in their intestines at birth. It should be passed within 24 hours of birth or it may cause blockage of the intestines. Colostrum, or early milk, is uniquely designed to help move this substance through and out of the infant's body.
- Formula feeding may increase the risk of sudden infant death syndrome (SIDS). According to the American Academy of Family Physicians, the special ingredients in breast milk lower your baby's risk of SIDS.
- Breast feeding makes vaccines work better.

Breast feeding helps mothers as well. After pregnancy, the uterus shrinks more quickly in women who breast-feed. Milk production also burns calories—about 500 a day. A natural hormone made during breast-feeding also has a calming effect on the mother. Not breast-feeding increases a mother's risk of breast cancer. Finally, breast-feeding decreases the chance of getting osteoporosis later in life.

Breast Feeding and Optimal Development of the Jaws, Teeth, and Face

Back in the 1920s when young mothers started to bottle-feed babies on the advice of their doctors, the problems all began! Instead of the natural sucking involved in breast-feeding, babies had to keep from choking on bottled milk by moving their tongues in ways that were not natural. The rubber nipples were more like a watering hose! The babies had to put their tongues in unnatural positions to stop milk coming in too fast or to get it in the right place to swallow when these artificial nipples were stuck in their mouths. Because these abnormal tongue movements were repeated, the wrong way became permanent. The baby's brain was programmed to send messages through the nerves to the muscles, getting them to move abnormally to try to cope with the bottle feeding.

The bottle-fed baby also swallows air—which is why you must stop often to burp a bottle-fed baby. Even after stopping the bottle, children continue to swallow air, which interferes with eating habits and digestion. The abnormal swallow that persists makes the tongue put unnatural forces on the teeth with each swallow. These forces actually push the teeth out of position. Often the result is the need for orthodontic work (braces) or painful temporomandibular joint (TMJ) problems (see chapter 12). Worst of all, this disruption caused by bottle feeding can lead to periodontal (gum) disease.

A normal swallow is when the tip of the tongue hits against the *rugae,* the little "tire treads" right behind the back of the front teeth inside the mouth. It should berth itself there and the body of the tongue should dump the liquid or food back. In abnormal or reverse swallow, the tip of the tongue goes against the teeth, and that causes mouth breathing, so that a lot of air is taken in, causing burping or spitting up.

Weak lip muscles and mouth breathing develop from the abnormal swallow, particularly while the child is asleep. This causes the mouth to be dry, which makes it more likely that plaque will form on the teeth. When the mouth dries, the bacteria grow. Many other problems in speech, digestion, and even the appearance of the face occur because of weak facial muscles.

Breast feeding helps the normal development of the mouth and face. Suckling at the breast requires the use of different muscles than does bottle feeding. When a baby breast-feeds, more energy is used, and the muscles around the mouth are used more efficiently in order to draw the nipple and much of the areola well back into the mouth. In this position, the nipple nestles against the junction of the hard and soft palates. You can feel this area where the hard part of the upper roof of the mouth becomes soft, back near the opening of the throat.

During this step in breast feeding, the infant's tongue moves up and forward to grasp the nipple as the gums compress the areola. The tongue moves backward to help deliver the milk. In a bottle-fed infant, the tongue is thrust against the nipple of the bottle to control the flow of milk. This action is easier to do and there is less muscular activity. Researchers have found that breast-fed children have a lower incidence and severity of misaligned teeth than bottle-fed babies. The longer the babies breast-fed, the lower was the chance of crooked teeth.

To prevent caries (cavities) in the infants it is important that milk does not "pool" around the teeth. The longer the milk remains in contact with the teeth, the higher is the risk of caries. During breast feeding, the position of the nipple back in the mouth makes it possible for the milk to be delivered past the area of the teeth, where the milk sugar can't do any harm. Other benefits of breast feeding include:

- Fewer cavities. Bottle-fed babies are at increased risk for "baby bottle caries" when put to bed with a bottle containing formula, milk, juice, or other fluids high in carbohydrates. Extensive dental repair may be needed at a cost of thousands of dollars.
- Better speech development. Tongue-thrust problems often develop among bottle-fed babies as they try to slow down the flow of milk coming from the artificial nipple. This can lead to speech problems, as well as mouth breathing, lip biting, gum disease, and a generally unattractive appearance.
- Better development of the airways in the nose and throat. This may prevent snoring later in life as well as sleep apnea (stopping breathing for short periods during sleeping).

Successful breast feeding doesn't come "naturally." It will help to discuss with your doctor the "how to" of the technique and how to prevent problems ahead of time. You can also get excellent breast feeding support from the La Leche League, an international organization dedicated to helping women have a good breast feeding experience (see Resource Section).

What to Eat When Breast Feeding

When you nurse your baby, you are the source of all the nutrients your newborn needs to grow and thrive. Good food choices will also help you regain your energy, health, and figure. Here are some simple guidelines:

- *Fruits and vegetables:* Each day, include at least five servings of fresh fruits and vegetables including at least one serving of a dark-orange vegetable (sweet potatoes, yams, acorn squash), two servings of dark-green leafy vegetables, and one serving of citrus fruit. For example, at breakfast eat a banana and a glass of fresh-squeezed orange juice or an orange (with other foods). For lunch, have a glass of tomato juice and a salad, and have at least a cup of vegetables with dinner.
- Grains: Have at least six servings of breads and cereals daily. These could include high-fiber cereal for breakfast, two slices of whole-grain bread for lunch in a sandwich, and brown rice or whole-wheat pasta at dinner.

NOTE: If you don't feel like eating a lot of food, make sure that what you do eat is of high quality, preferably organic. If you don't want to do much cooking, you can get quick-cooking organic oatmeal, and whole-grain organic dry cereals, breads, and crackers.

- *Milk:* You need the calcium that is in at least four glasses of fat-free or low-fat milk daily. You can also get calcium from plain yogurt and low-fat cheeses. For women who are lactose intolerant, calcium-fortified soy milk or calcium-fortified orange juice can help meet the requirements, but calcium supplements may be needed. These should always contain magnesium since magnesium, prevents the constipating effects that sometimes occur with calcium-only supplements. A pregnant woman should get 1,500 mg a day of calcium and half that amount of magnesium. Remember, that supplements are not a substitute for a poor diet—they help you get the most benefit from your food.

- *Protein:* Include three daily servings of lean meats, eggs, chicken, fish, or cooked dried beans or peas. The more you can eat of organic, hormone-free protein sources, the better. You won't have to detoxify pesticides and hormones, and neither will your baby.

- Take a multiple vitamin and mineral supplement that has at least 100% of the U.S. Recommended Dietary Allowances (RDA). Make sure it contains 400 mg of folic acid since this key vitamin will be depleted during nursing.

- *Beverages:* Remember that whatever you drink, your nursing baby drinks, also. So drink lots of water and avoid alcohol and caffeine from coffee, tea, and soft drinks. Caffeine in breast milk can interfere with your baby's sleeping patterns.

- Balance your calories. While nursing you need an additional 500 calories a day over your prepregnancy requirement. Your vitamin and mineral needs are even higher than they were during pregnancy, so every bite must be full of nutrients. This will ensure the best health for your baby. Nursing is not the time to diet or skip meals! Your body is still in a "calorie-storing" model to ensure that you have enough nutrients to produce healthy milk for your baby.

- Be prepared. Babies take up a lot of your time. But you need to eat regularly, so plan ahead. Stock the kitchen, the refrigerator, your glove compartment in the car, and your purse with healthful foods and snacks.

A hint of garlic may whet a baby's appetite. Researchers at the Monell Chemical Senses Center in Philadelphia found that babies seemed to prefer garlicky milk, remaining attached to the breast for longer periods after their mothers took garlic capsules. In contrast, when mothers drank alcohol-spiked juice, infants drank significantly less milk.

Again, we recommend that you enlist the aid of your doctor in helping you to prepare for breast feeding. Not all doctors are interested in this subject, but he or she may recommend someone who can help. One doctor says that the recent decline in breast feeding results from efforts to promote breast feeding without giving the practical help women need. Physicians as well as others assume that this is just a natural process and that women know how to do it. Many women end up frustrated and angry and give up. Common hospital practices such as separating mother and infant and feeding formula to infants in the nursery undermine new mothers' efforts to breast feed. Shorter hospital stays are making the problem worse, reducing the opportunities for breast-feeding education and sending mothers home before their milk has had time to come in. Interviews with 392 women in a maternity ward that switched to "baby-friendly" rules found that 63% of newborns were allowed to breast feed in the first hour of life, only 30% were given foods other than breast milk, and 82% of mothers received instruction in breast feeding. As a result, more women were still nursing 2 months later. Another study found that pumped breast milk remained safe for 24 hours when stored at 59° F and 4 hours at 77° F, room temperature.

How do you know your baby is getting enough breast milk? According to the American Academy of Family Physicians, you know your baby is getting enough milk if:

- Your baby has at least six to eight wet diapers every day
- Your baby is back up to birth weight by 2 weeks of age
- You can hear your baby swallowing while breast feeding
- Your milk leaks from one breast when you are feeding the baby on the other breast
- Your baby has four or more bowel movements every day

To be successful, nursing must follow birth as quickly as possible. This first nursing empties the milk ducts of colostrum, the early milk, and reduces pressure in the breast. The colostrum is good for the baby—it contains many protective antibodies against viruses and bacteria. Even if a mother decides not to breast feed, she should at least let the baby have the colostrum.

What Gets into Breast Milk?

Many harmful substances can get into breast milk from the mother's diet or environment. Several studies showed that dental amalgam mercury from the mother's mouth could get into breast milk and build up in the tissues of unborn babies. Therefore, researchers did not think it was a good idea to put mercury-containing fillings in women's mouths before and during the childbearing age.

Removing mercury-containing fillings exposes unborn or newborn nursing babies to high levels of toxic mercury. Pregnancy is definitely *not* the time to have mercury fillings put in or removed.

Is there anything other than removal of amalgam fillings that could protect the unborn child from the toxic effects of mercury? One very effective nutrient is vitamin C. Vitamin C is a natural chelator of heavy metals such as mercury. Being a chelator means that vitamin C will wrap itself around the mercury and help push it out of the body. So every woman with mercury fillings who is about to conceive or who is pregnant should have a good intake of vitamin C to help reduce the body's levels of this toxic metal.

When Breast Feeding Is Not an Option

There are many reasons why a woman may choose not to breast-feed:

- Previous difficulty with breast feeding or knowing someone who had problems
- Being discouraged or embarrassed during early attempts that failed
- Lack of the milk ejection (letdown) reflex (can be inhibited by pain, anxiety, stress or smoking)
- Work-related factors; not all companies will allow time to use a breast pump or will have storage facilities for the milk
- Psychological reasons having to do with modesty, upbringing, husband's feelings about nursing, and so on
- Encouragement by family or friends not to breast feed: "it will ruin your figure"

- Lack of support from health professionals not trained or interested in helping
- Breast reduction or enlargement surgery that may interfere with nursing
- Taking antibiotics or medications that may harm the baby
- Having an infectious disease such as hepatitis or the HIV virus

Whatever the reasons, a woman who chooses not to breast-feed needs to make the right choices about bottle nipples and commercial formulas. The choice of nipple is especially important for the baby's future dental health.

Bottle Feeding and Choosing the Right Nipple

Most artificial nipples are not designed to encourage the normal growth and development of a child's face and teeth. Bottle feeding with a conventional nipple forces the tongue, lips, and jaws into an abnormal position. This can cause the muscles that move them to develop out of balance with one another, leading to malocclusion (teeth out of line). There are three important factors in nipple design that every mother should know before choosing a nipple for her child's bottle: length, flexibility, and flow.

Length. Length is very important because the wrong length can prevent normal growth of the mouth and may disfigure the baby's growing face. When an infant is born, the lower face has reached only 40% of its adult size. During the first year, the baby's face will increase in size and also grow downward and forward. The type of bone at the top of the mouth is soft. Any force placed on it easily changes its shape. The wrong length of nipple could change the direction of growth or the shape of the face during this growth period.

During breast feeding, studies have shown that the mother's nipple is made so that it can fit into the baby's mouth. The nipple can then increase by about half an inch in length during nursing.

Artificial nipples are 1.2 to 2.1 times larger than the nursing mother's nipple, and they keep their length during feeding. This large nipple is used for babies with faces of all different sizes, so the baby must adapt to the artificial nipple. In breast feeding, the baby's tongue elongates the mother's nipple to the proper length for that infant's mouth and places it against the top of its mouth with the tongue underneath. With the long artificial nipple, the position of the baby's tongue is very different. The shape of the nipple makes it impossible for the baby to hold its tongue underneath the nipple and press the nipple against the hard palate in the roof of the mouth. Also, the shape of the nipple itself forces the baby's lips into a rounded position, causing a weakening of the lip muscles and forcing the tongue to move in a forward movement rather than in a backward movement during nursing. Thus, the wrong length of nipple can interfere with the normal facial and dental growth. So a mother using an artificial nipple must try to find one that is best suited for her child's size and rate of facial growth.

Out of 985 patients in one study, examined and found to have abnormal (deviate) swallowing patterns, 700 of these children were bottle fed using long nipples. Another 150 were bottle-fed for the first 3 months. Only 60 children who were breast-fed (only until 4 months of age) had swallowing problems. Of children who were breast fed completely, 75 had swallowing problems, but all of these got a fast flow of milk from their mothers' breasts. These results lead to one conclusion, that the way a baby nurses plays a significant role in the development of abnormal mouth and facial muscle balance.

Flexibility. The second important factor in choosing a nipple is the flexibility of the nipple design. It needs to be flexible enough so that it can be shaped in the baby's mouth, with the tongue moving easily. Also, the hole in the nipple must be designed so that the milk will not flow too fast or too slow. The flexibility will allow the baby to nurse with lips closed, rather than held in the rounded position with lips open. The open-lip position can result in weak lip muscles and a habit of mouth breathing. Dental authorities have long recognized that strong facial muscles play an important role in the normal development and growth of the face and eruption of the teeth.

Flow. The rate of flow of milk into the baby's mouth will be controlled by the action of the baby's tongue. In breast feeding, the nipple is held against the top of the baby's mouth, and there is a rhythmic rocking back and forth of the tongue to control the flow of milk. Except for the initial letdown of the mother's milk, the flow from the breast is controlled by the baby's sucking and breathing. The tongue acts as a regulator valve, preventing overflow by pressing against and releasing the nipple. A good artificial nursing system should act the same way as the natural nipple.

Mothers should understand that anything placed in the mouth with force against the soft bones of the top of the mouth acts like an orthodontic appliance (braces). It affects the way that the face and the teeth will develop. In this case, teeth will be pushed out of line. So choose nipples with care and with the above three factors in mind: length, flexibility, and flow.

There is a nipple designed to allow the baby to nurse as if from the breast. It was originally called the Nuk-Sauger nipple. Now it is just called Nuk® and is sold by the Gerber Products Company (see Resources). The shape of the Nuk is quite different from conventional nipples: a large bulb at the base and a much smaller bulb at the tip. The baby must work to get the milk from the nipple just as he or she would from the breast. A baby used to a conventional nipple and its easy milk flow could have some difficulty getting used to it. Some parents may not like the fact that it takes longer to feed with the Nuk or that it is more difficult to properly fit the Nuk to the bottle. Dr. Jerome Mittelman believes that Nuk nipples are anatomically correct—that they have a shape very similar to natural nipples. Jean Barilla was told by her daughter that the only artificial nipples her children would accept were Nuk nipples. These children were breast fed for at least 1 year before switching to a bottle. Information on Nuk pacifiers is found in chapter 4.

In December of 1998, the Gerber company voluntarily recalled all of its soft vinyl infant care and toy products intended for mouth contact. They did this because the products contained chemical softening ingredients called phthalates. Since the U.S. Consumer Product Safety Commission had concerns about the safety of this chemical for babies, the company took the products off the market. The Gerber Company noted that their leading Nuk® line of teethers, pacifiers, and nipples are completely phthalate-free.

All About Formula

No formula could really duplicate breast milk. "We're always discovering things in human milk that are there in small quantities that hadn't been looked at before," says John C. Wallingford, Ph.D., an infant nutrition specialist with the FDA's Center for Food Safety and Applied Nutrition. It will be a very long time, possibly never, before mother's milk is copied exactly in a laboratory.

Homemade formulas should not be used, according to the FDA. Cow's milk doesn't have all of the nutrients in the right amounts needed for your baby's health. Substituting evaporated milk for whole milk may make formula easier to digest, but it is poor nutrition when compared to commercially prepared formula. According to FDA regulations, the following nutrients must be in all formulas: protein, fat, linoleic acid, vitamin A, vitamin D, vitamin E, vitamin K, thiamine (vitamin B_1), riboflavin (vitamin B_2), vitamin B_{12}, vitamin B_6 (pyridoxine), niacin (vitamin B_3), folic acid, copper, iodine, sodium, potassium, and chloride. In addition, formulas *not* made from cow's milk must include biotin, choline, and inositol.

Soy "milk" sold in health food stores and supermarkets is *not* the same as soy formula that is used for babies with milk (lactose) intolerance. Use of soy milk or soy drinks can actually be life-threatening for the baby that drinks one of these in place of formula. Key nutrients are missing from soy beverages. Because of the danger that parents may think that a beverage labeled "soy milk" is appropriate to feed an infant, many makers of these products have put a warning message on the label: "Do Not Use As Infant Formula." The FDA, however, does not have the regulatory authority to require this warning. So be sure a soy milk is okay for feeding to your baby—ask your doctor or other health professional about any soy or other non-cow based milk that you choose.

What Should Formula Contain?

In 1998, the Life Sciences Research Office of the American Society for Nutritional Sciences, Bethesda, Maryland, released a report recommending what nutrients should be present in commercial formulas. The report was cosponsored by the Health Protection Branch of Health Canada and is based on evaluations by an expert panel of people from over 263 organizations. The recommendations are as follows:

Essential fats (linoleic acid, alpha-linolenic acid)
Carbohydrate
Protein
Amino acids (carnitine, taurine)
Nucleotides
Choline and inositol
Minerals (calcium, phosphorus, magnesium, iron, zinc, manganese, copper, iodine, sodium, potassium, chloride, selenium, fluoride)
Vitamins (A, C, D, E, K, thiamine, riboflavin, niacin, pyridoxine, cobalamin (B_{12}), folic acid, pantothenic acid, biotin)

The panel did not recommend adding polyunsaturated fatty acids (arachidonic acid, AA, and docosahexanoic acid, DHA). They decided to wait for 5 years until the next review to make a decision. These essential fats are discussed in chapter X. Even though they knew that these important fats are lower in the blood of formula-fed babies than for breast-fed babies, they felt there wasn't enough evidence to include them. These fats are found in high amounts in the retina of the eye and in the brain, and there is good evidence that babies with a good supply of these fats have better learning skills.

Here is additional information on the components of formula.

Carbohydrate (sugar). Lactose (milk sugar) accounts for 40% of the sugar in cow's-milk-based formulas just as it does in breast milk. If an infant has lactose intolerance (due to a lack of or low level of the liver enzyme lactase), lactose-free soy-based formulas may be used. The carbohydrates in soy-based formulas include sucrose, glucose polymers (corn syrup solids), and cornstarch, which are easily absorbed by the lactose-intolerant baby.

Fats. Infants need fat in their diet. Because infants drink only a small amount of fluid each day, the fluid must contain as many nutrients as possible. Fat provides the highest number of calories (more than double those of carbohydrates and protein), and babies need calories.

Over half the calories in formula and in breast milk come from fat. Both breast milk and formula contain 20 calories per ounce and 30 grams of fat per liter of milk. But the similarities stop there. Formulas add fat in the form of palm, coconut, corn, soy, or safflower oils. These formula fats are very different from the healthy, natural fats found in mother's milk. Another advantage of breast milk is that you won't have to worry about fats becoming rancid (spoiled) if they come directly from the breast.

Protein. Protein is the most important factor for proper growth and development of a baby. Most infant formulas contain 15 grams of protein per liter (human milk contains 10–12 grams per liter during early breast feeding and 9-12 grams during later breast feeding). Because cow's milk is low in taurine and cysteine compared to breast milk, these are often added to formulas. Taurine and cysteine are important in brain function and for regulating the growth of cells and the membranes around cells.

The type of protein in formula is an area of major controversy. Human milk is composed of 65% whey protein and 35% casein protein. Whey from human milk contains such vital substances as alpha-lactalbumin, lactoferrin, immunoglobulins, albumin, enzymes, growth factors, and hormones. In contrast, cow's milk contains only 18% whey versus 82% casein. Cow's milk contains beta-globulin, of unknown function, and other proteins that are destroyed during commercial heat processing. These heated formula proteins do not provide any immunity and their ability to cause allergies is increased.

Vitamins and Minerals.   All the required vitamins and minerals were listed above (page 48). If you look at these nutrients in formula, the amounts are adequate for infant nutrition. In fact, formula could be a better choice than breast milk, if a mother is eating a diet that makes her milk deficient in some of these nutrients. A woman on an inadequate diet may produce breast milk poor in vitamins B_6, B_{12}, and folic acid. Strict vegetarians who breast-feed and do not take supplemental B_6 produce milk that contains little or none of this vitamin. If a mother's breast milk is deficient in any vitamins or minerals, the doctor should recommend dietary supplements for the baby. In such cases, formula may be a better choice.

When we discussed iron above (in the breast milk section) it was noted that infants absorb all the iron in breast milk, but cannot absorb all the iron in infant formulas. Some parents believe that in prepared formula, iron causes stomach discomfort, constipation, diarrhea, colic, and irritability. In response, some manufacturers have marketed low-iron formulas containing only 2 milligrams of iron per liter of formula. The low-iron formulas may alleviate these symptoms, but will not provide enough iron for blood formation and should be avoided. Adding some acidophilus powder to the formula or a half teaspoon of plain, organic yogurt will help with such digestive problems.

Nucleotides.   These nutrients are the building blocks of RNA and DNA (the genetic material). They occur naturally in breast milk and are necessary for normal body function. Nucleotides are necessary for cells to grow and increase in number, which is important to infant growth and development. The nucleotides are adenylic acid, guanylic acid, cytidylic acid, and uridylic acid.

Never use a microwave oven to prepare or warm formula. The milk may heat unevenly, resulting in "hot spots" that can seriously burn your baby. Also, it has been reported in the *Lancet,* a major medical journal, that microwaving baby formula made from cow's milk can convert the amino acid proline present in the milk to a toxic form. If this unnatural amino acid is used to build proteins in the baby's body, it "can lead to structural, functional, and immunological changes." Heating formula on the stove doesn't cause this change.

When preparing formula, be very careful about the water used to dilute concentrated formula. Old water pipes can leach lead into the water. There is more lead in hot water pipes than in cold. When a faucet is first turned on in the morning, the lead content is higher—so let the water run for a few minutes. Good quality bottled water is recommended if you are not sure about the water pipes. Boiling the water won't help because this will only concentrate the lead.

Most manufacturers of infant formula provide directions for mixing their products with water and usually do not specify any type of water except for saying that the water should be safe to drink. In most cases, it is safe to mix formula using ordinary cold tap water that has run for at least 2 minutes and has been boiled for 1 minute. Some water companies sell water that is labeled for use in preparing infant formula. This water must meet the same standards for tap water as established by the Environmental Protection Agency. The label must also state that the bottle water is not sterile and should also be boiled for 1 minute before mixing with infant formula.

Excess fluoride in the water used to make formula can also be toxic. See chapter 10 for more information including "A Mother's Sad Story."

Baby Bottle Tooth Decay

In any place where there are parents pushing around babies and toddlers in carriages or strollers, many of these children can be seen drinking constantly from bottles containing anything from milk to soda. Many of these same children are put to bed with a bottle. This can have serious consequences for their dental health.

Johns Hopkins University in Baltimore explained the link between the wrong way to bottle-feed and tooth decay. According to Johns Hopkins, millions of American parents put their infants and toddlers to bed each night with a bottle, often containing juice or some other sugary drink. It may help settle the children down, but for years dentists have tried to stop the practice. They argue that sugar in the drink helps bacteria grow in the mouth and contributes to the serious problem of baby bottle tooth decay (BBTD). How bad the decay gets depends on what is in the bottle as well as how often it's done and for how long the bottle is in the baby's mouth.

This risk of potentially devastating dental decay exists not only for the bottle-fed child; it can happen with the breast-fed child as well. Keeping the baby nursing for long periods of time and letting erupted teeth be exposed to breast milk lactose (a sugar) without the correct oral hygiene measures will produce the same decay in bottle- or breast-fed babies.

Recently, some experts have argued that plain old milk is the best bottle filler at night because it lacks the sugars that can destroy a child's first set of teeth. But Johns Hopkins visiting dental professor Dr. Elliott Schwartz isn't so sure that milk is the answer, either. "Ideally, if you're going to put the child to sleep with a bottle, it should be a bottle containing water and just that, just water. No sugar within the water, no other carbohydrates within the water," explains Schwartz. "Everything else contains sugar. Even juices contain sugars and natural carbohydrates." But no matter what goes into the bottle, dental experts agree that parents should try to wean their little ones off a regular bottle starting at about age 1.

According to the American Academy of Pediatric Dentistry, (AAPD), a bottle containing anything but water exposes your infant or child to the danger of developing BBTD. Pacifiers dipped in sugar or honey are just as dangerous to your baby's teeth. When a child sleeps, the production of saliva, which protects teeth from bacteria that cause tooth decay, slows down. This lack of saliva allows liquids remaining in the mouth to pool around the sleeping child's teeth. Sugars in the liquid combine with bacteria in the mouth to form acid that dissolves the immature enamel. Newly erupted first teeth are highly susceptible to decay. Unfortunately, it does not take long for extensive tooth decay to develop. BBTD is easy to prevent. The following AAPD recommendations will help your child avoid this painful condition:

1. Infants should not be put to sleep with a bottle containing a liquid other than water at bedtime.
2. Once the first primary tooth begins to erupt, stop "on demand" breast feeding at night.
3. Have infants drink from a cup as they approach their first

birthday—between 9 and 12 months old. Wean them from the bottle at 12–14 months of age.

4. Drinking juices from a bottle should be avoided. When juices are offered it should be from a cup.

5. Start oral hygiene measures by the time the first primary tooth erupts. Massage and cleanse your infant's gums with a very clean soft cloth or piece of sterile gauze after each feeding. Your pediatric dentist can demonstrate the best position and technique. (See pages 75–76 for details).

6. Schedule a visit to the dentist within 6 months of eruption of the first tooth. The first visit will focus on prevention, teaching, and any questions you may have. This is similar to a well-baby visit with your pediatrician.

7. Since you are not the only person who cares for your child, warn grandparents and anyone else who cares for your baby or child about the hazards of putting him or her to sleep with bottles and sweetened pacifiers.

Dr. Arthur Alban, a pedodontist (children's dentist) in Riverside, California, says that apple juice in a bottle has a particularly bad effect on teeth. He tells of a case where a parent brought in a child for an examination because the child, who was old enough to have several teeth, did not have any yet. Dr. Alban found that several teeth had actually erupted, but had rapidly decayed down to the gum line.

Shachi D. Shantinath, D.D.S., and colleagues, studied parents of children with nursing caries and parents whose children were caries-free. They found that the two groups differed most in the use of feeding to assist with sleep. Parents of children with caries were more likely to have fed the child in response to crying or waking, given a bottle to help children fall asleep at night, and fed children at nap time. The parents of caries-free children weaned them from the breast or bottle an average of 6 months earlier than the caries group. Although children should certainly not be put to bed with a bottle containing anything but water, if the child needs a bottle before going to sleep as part of his feeding, you need to wipe the mouth—the gums and whatever teeth have come in—with a damp gauze or cloth.

Parents may turn to feeding to help their child because feeding is usually effective in calming the child. But there are other ways of calming children more protective of the teeth. Many infants and toddlers have sleep problems that can make it rough for weary parents. Having bedtime routines (bedtime at the same hour, story reading, and so on) can help decrease sleep problems and reduce the need for sleep-associated feeding that can lead to nursing caries. Nursing mothers need to avoid stimulants that can get into breast milk such as caffeine from coffee, tea, or chocolate. The caffeine will make it difficult for the baby to sleep. Holding and cuddling, without feeding, may also help.

The sound of a heartbeat has been shown to be soothing to babies, supposedly because it's like being in the womb. There are sound machines that you can buy that produce the sound of a heartbeat or other soothing sounds. Some have colored lights along with the sound that can also soothe a restless infant. Some babies may also respond to aromatherapy scents in the air, such as lavender, known for its relaxing properties.

When to Wean and How

There is no proof that beginning solid foods early results in more rapid growth of your baby. There is a good case for not weaning early. According to Betty Kamen, Ph.D, a noted nutritionist, adding other foods to the diet of a 4- to-6-month-old nursing infant may result in less iron being absorbed. The longer babies are breast-fed, the lower are their cholesterol readings as teenagers or young adults. Another reason for not introducing foods too early is that the enzyme ptyalin, present in saliva, cannot work properly until 1 year of age. This enzyme helps digest starches such as those found in cereals and vegetables.

Late Bottle Weaning

Many mothers, particularly those that work, continue to bottle-feed their children beyond age 2, thus increasing the risk of dental caries and overweight later in life. Dr. Lawrence D. Hammer and colleagues at Stanford University in Palo Alto, California, found that 42% of infants continued to receive bottle-feeds beyond 2 years of age and 16% beyond 3 years. They were surprised to find these figures in well-educated, middle-class mothers.

Slow weaning is a good way to start introducing solid foods. If the baby is still drinking breast milk, the mother's own food antibodies in her milk will boost the baby's immune response to the new food. Breast-fed babies have fewer food allergies as a result.

After hearing the pros and cons of breast and bottle feeding, we hope that you can make an informed decision about what to feed your baby. Since the benefits of breast feeding by far outweigh those of bottle feeding, please try to breast-feed your new baby.

CHAPTER 4

Sucking, Thumb Sucking, and Pacifiers

Even before birth, a baby's need to suck is very strong. You can look at your baby's first picture—with ultrasound—and see the thumb sucking for yourself! As with most mammals, the newborn's life depends on its ability to suckle. If it cannot latch on tightly and suck hard enough, it will die. Babies are also born with a "rooting" reflex. Did you ever notice that, when either side of a newborn's mouth is touched, it turns its head toward that side? This reflex allows the newborn to find the nipple.

Sucking is also a reflex. When an object is placed in the newborn's mouth, sucking begins immediately. These rooting and sucking reflexes allow a baby to start nursing immediately after birth. If the baby is not placed at the mother's breast in the delivery room, feedings are usually started within 4 hours after birth—the earlier, the better.

Why Stop Thumb Sucking?

Thumb sucking or finger sucking is a habit that many infants have difficulty giving up. This habit may cause your child to develop a malformed palate (roof of the mouth) and crooked baby teeth. These will cause problems a long time before the permanent teeth come in. These problems come from pressure applied by the thumb on the teeth and roof of the mouth.

How bad the problem will be depends on how often and how long the thumb is sucked, as well as the position in which the thumb is placed in the mouth. The lineup between the upper and lower jaws may also be affected. Speech defects can occur because of teeth that do not line up properly as a result of thumb sucking or finger sucking.

Thumb, finger, and pacifier sucking (if it's the wrong type of pacifier) all affect the teeth essentially the same way—negatively.

The Importance of the Tongue

The tongue has an important relationship with the palate and the teeth. If the baby sucks on poorly designed artificial nipples, it can affect the development of normal tongue movement and cause abnormal facial muscle actions. The open-lip position necessary for bottle feeding can result in weak lip muscles and the habit of mouth breathing. These problems associated with bottle feeding, together with the effects on teeth from thumb sucking, will set the stage for future visits to the orthodontist (see chapter 12). Breast feeding can therefore be thought of as "preventive orthodontics."

The Palatal Arch and Tooth Development

About 8½ weeks after conception, the palatal arch forms in the fetus. If the mother's diet has been poor, this arch will not develop completely. So even at this early stage, the future health and well-being of the baby have already been set by the mother's nutritional state.

When the palatal arch is well formed, crooked teeth are less likely to form in the future. A correctly formed palatal arch encourages the tongue to rest in the normal position against the ridges on the roof of the mouth. This is important because the normal position helps the continued normal development of the arch. If the tongue is down in the bottom of the mouth (where it will be with thumb sucking), the arch doesn't develop properly and can lead to incorrect swallowing. As discussed earlier, both incorrect breast feeding or bottle feeding can cause incorrect swallowing.

When the tongue is correctly placed on the rugae behind the front teeth, proper swallowing will follow, reducing tooth alignment problems. Normal tongue placement will also result in nasal breathing, the right type of breathing.

When the palate is correctly formed, the temporomandibular joint (TMJ), which joins the upper and lower jaw just in front of the ear, will function normally. This may help avoid future TMJ problems, such as pain.

A correctly formed palatal arch also encourages normal development of the bones and muscles in the face responsible for the ability to smile. Poor development of the bones results in inadequate pull of those muscles attached to the bones, including the major muscle that enables us to smile. That nice smile that goes with those nice teeth also depends on tongue actions.

Tongue displacement also causes swallowing difficulties. In a normal swallow, the tip of your tongue braces on the rugae, the little bumps on the roof of your mouth just behind your upper front teeth. The tongue then propels the food back and down. In the abnormal swallow, the tip may move to the right, forward, left, or even brace itself against the lower teeth. There are many variations. Often the body of the tongue slips in between the back teeth.

These problems have been called *traumatic swallow* because they have traumatic effects on the teeth and jaws. In fact, one study showed that 74% of people with poor teeth alignment have such problems. And it all starts with bottle feeding.

First, the baby's tongue must push against the nipple to keep from choking. Second, the incorrect shape of the artificial nipple makes the problem worse. Third, bottle-fed babies swallow air along with the milk, which is why they need "burping."

About 10% of breast-feeding mothers have "fast-flowing" milk that can create similar problems. Such feedings (bottle or fast flow) repeated over and over create a neuromuscular (nerve and muscle) pattern that becomes subconscious for the child. From then on, throughout life, these children will have an abnormal swallow.

How can you tell if you or your children have it? An informed dentist or myofunctional therapist (see Resources) can make the diagnosis for you. But if you have a problem swallowing pills or vita-

mins, or if you sleep with your mouth open, this may be a good indication that you need help.

Abnormal Tongue Movement

Abnormal tongue movement can push a tooth, much as an orthodontist does with braces, and move a tooth out of its proper position. With each abnormal swallow, tongue pressures can be
measured in pounds. When repeated thousands of times a day, the
result is a bad bite that can lead to clenching the jaws and grinding
the teeth. One result of these actions can be TMJ headaches. If the
teeth are adjusted to help resolve the TMJ problem, in a short time,
the tongue will again push the teeth out of position. This also explains why when orthodontists remove braces, the teeth sometimes
move out of position. The dentist must then try a retainer to realign
the teeth.

Gum problems can also result from abnormal tongue movement. In abnormal swallow cases, we often find flaccid (limp) lips
and mouth breathing, particularly while asleep. This dries out the
saliva, allowing the plaque germs to breed in the dry environment
and inflame the gums.

Dentists will use peroxide and antibiotics, and periodontists will
use antibiotics and surgery—but almost all of them look right past
the tongue since they are not trained in corrective measures. What
can be done to keep your child's gums healthy? The best thing you
can do is to prevent the problem in the first place. Breast-feed your
baby! If you can't breast-feed, make sure you get the right artificial
nipple. In the past, some orthodontists recognized the problem.
They gave their patients (children and adults) a few exercises to do.
But they still had abnormal swallows. Why? This was because people could learn to swallow correctly when they thought about it.
But as soon as they stopped thinking about it, the tongue went right
back to its old habits. Only treatment by a competent myofunctional therapist will completely correct the problem. That's why it is
better not to start the wrong habit to begin with.

In addition to having gum problems and being cavity-prone because of dry mouths, children with tongue problems can also have

eating problems. Swallowing a lot of air can give them stomach distress. Children without these problems chew their food more thoroughly before swallowing. They also may have to drink less liquid with their meals, since they have a wetter mouth (from not mouth breathing). Too much liquid during eating dilutes stomach acid, and food cannot be digested as well. Bowel movements become more normal and regular after treatment. Older patients find that they can swallow pills after treatment.

The Tongue and Speech

Abnormal tongue movements can also affect speech. The facial muscles used in swallowing and chewing are the same ones used in speech. When these muscles are not functioning properly, speech may be affected. Speech may be slow, sluggish, and "mushy" sounding. The words and sounds may be imprecise and slurred. There may be difficulties in pronouncing certain sounds such as *sh*, *ch*, *s*, *z*, and others when there is incorrect tongue position and swallowing. Conventional speech therapy doesn't take care of these problems. Correcting the speech sounds without fixing the facial muscle imbalance is not really getting to the cause. People who have had speech therapy often fall into old habits of pronunciation when excited or stressed, because the cause of the problem hasn't really been corrected.

Only a speech therapist who has been trained in myofunctional therapy will reposition the tongue and strengthen the facial muscles as well as treat the speech problems. Although it's good that these problems can be corrected, it's much better for the baby and parents to avoid having to seek help in the first place. Some of the ways to prevent the problems follow.

Pacifiers

Children should be encouraged to chew and bite as soon as possible—even before the first tooth comes into the mouth. It is important for tooth and facial development that you choose the right pacifier as discussed below. If your child does use a pacifier, please take precautions to ensure your child's safety:

- Never tie a pacifier around a baby's neck. The U.S. Consumer Product Safety Commission regularly receives reports of strangulation deaths involving pacifiers tied around a child's neck.
- Select a pacifier with sturdy, one-piece construction, made of nontoxic, flexible material, with an easily grasped handle such as the Nuk Orthodontic Pacifier. While we don't usually recommend specific products, in this case, the Nuk pacifiers and nipples are the only ones that meet the criteria for developmentally safe nursing aids.
- The pacifier should be too large to swallow (choose the right size), have a shield or mouth guard that can't be separated from the nipple, and have two ventilation holes.
- To ensure that a piece of the nipple can't break off in the baby's mouth, the nipple should be intact without holes or tears. Parents should pull on the nipple to test it, and replace the pacifier when the nipple shows signs of wear.

Questions Parents Ask About Thumb Sucking

Here are some questions parents ask and the American Association of Pediatric Dentistry's responses:

Q: Are these sucking habits bad for the teeth and jaws?

A: Most children stop sucking on thumbs, pacifiers, or other objects on their own between 2 and 4 years of age. They may stop a pacifier earlier if allowed to suck all they want. However, some children repeatedly suck on a finger, pacifier, or other object over long periods of time. In these children, the upper front teeth may tip toward the lip or not come in properly.

Q: What can I do to stop my child's habit?

A: Most children stop sucking habits on their own, but some children need the help of their parents and their pediatric dentist. When your child is old enough to understand the possible results of a sucking habit, your pediatric dentist can encourage your child to stop, as well as talk about what happens to the teeth if your child doesn't stop. This advice, coupled with support from parents, helps most children quit. If this approach doesn't work, your pediatric dentist may recommend a mouth appliance that blocks sucking habits.

Q: Are pacifiers a safer habit for the teeth than thumbs or fingers?

A: Thumb, finger, and [the wrong type of] pacifier all affect the teeth essentially the same way.

The Nuk Orthodontic Pacifier (see Resource section) not only is safer than thumb and finger, but is actually desirable. This is because the nipple part of the Nuk is shaped to hold the baby's tongue in a natural position, just as with the breast. The pacifier acts as a training device to prevent tongue thrusting and is used for early treatment of open bite and other simple orthodontic problems. It comes in three sizes: infants, birth to 6 months old, 6–18 month-old babies, and children 18 months to 3 years of age. The last one can be used to help prevent thumb sucking. Instead of trying to fight your child's need to suck, providing a pacifier that is actually good for your baby is a better solution.

How to Break the Habit

There are many suggestions for breaking the thumb-sucking habit. Some are more "friendly" than others.We believe that prevention is the best method of avoiding future problems. If you can get your newborn to prefer the right type of pacifier to thumb sucking or finger sucking, it will be an easier habit to break later on. While continued use of the wrong pacifier can lead to similar problems as thumb sucking, the right pacifier actually benefits the baby.

The timing of treatment is very important. If your child is not willing to give up thumb sucking, wait awhile and try again—there shouldn't be a "stop right now" attitude on the part of the parent.

Reminders such as a Band-Aid on the thumb (especially those with pictures) can help. An "all or nothing" approach is not necessary. You can offer rewards (a gold star on a chart, dimes, an extra bedtime story) for days when your child is successful. Praise your child when he or she is successful. Take one step at a time. For example, you could encourage your child not to suck during one day-time activity, like story time or television watching. Gradually add another activity until daytime sucking is controlled.

Once daytime sucking is controlled, you can help your child to give up the sucking habit during sleep. Since the child is sleepy and can't respond to encouragement, you may have to use an aid such as a glove, sock, or thumb/finger guard to help stop the habit.

The American Dental Association advises:

- Parents should reward the child when he or she refrains from thumb sucking.
- If other positive approaches such as encouragement do not work, parents can bandage the child's thumb at night or place a sock over it to prevent the child from thumb sucking.
- Talk to your dentist about methods that may help your child break his or her thumb-sucking habit.

Natural and More Humane Teething and Thumb-Sucking Remedies

Trying to stop a thumb-sucking problem by force or nagging can be traumatic—for you and your child. And often, it doesn't work. Fortunately, there are comfortable, effective methods for parents to use in helping children kick the habit. The Nuk pacifier, if used early and freely, may prevent the problem in the first place. There are videos such as *Mr. Wizard's Thumb's Out,* produced by a speech pathologist and myofunctional therapist, Linda Bejoian, M.S. It motivates children with an excellent program for overcoming the habit (see Resources). *My Thumb and I* is a book by Carol Mayer, M.S., also a speech pathologist and orofacial myologist. It's written for children 6 to 10 years old. There are guidelines for parents and fun activities for the child (see Resources).

Teething can be a very trying time for both baby and parents. Even the most tranquil baby can become a terror when teething—with good reason. The pain can be constant and excruciating. The first sign that Baby is starting to go through the teething process is usually excessive drooling and restlessness. The baby's gums become red and swollen, possibly even blistered where the new tooth is coming in. And most children become cranky or clingy, sometimes refusing to eat or sleep. A fever, a cold, diarrhea, rashes on the face, or ear, nose, and throat infections may accompany these symptoms. These infections may happen because a break in the gums made by the cutting tooth allows germs to get into the baby's system.

Painkillers are not the answer. Teething biscuits (those not made with sugar) and frozen teething rings may work to some extent, but babies need plenty of comfort and love at this time as well as help from natural ways to curb the pain and soothe the irritability. Here are some suggestions:

Apple: Unsulfured dried apple rings are a tasty alternative to conventional teething rings. They can be kept in the freezer until use.

Carrot: A frozen carrot makes a good natural teething aid. Chewing offers some relief, and the cold eases swelling and tenderness. As the carrot is chewed, it dissolves in the baby's mouth.

Chamomile: Chamomile oil can be rubbed directly on the baby's gums and is soothing as well as calming.

Clove: A few drops of clove oil can be diluted in a tablespoon of olive oil and rubbed onto the baby's gums. Never use it full strength; it may inflame the gums.

Garlic: Garlic oil can be applied directly to the gums or mixed with olive oil. The antibacterial properties of garlic will decrease the possibility of infection in the open gums.

Other hints:

- Press your finger or knuckles gently against the baby's gums. Dunking your finger in icy water first will be even more soothing.
- Keep a small metal spoon in the freezer. Hold it against the baby's gums. NOTE: Do not take the frozen spoon from the freezer and instantly put it on your baby's gums. Some freezers are cold enough to cause the metal to stick to the skin.
- A damp, clean washcloth, kept in the freezer, can be given to the baby to chomp on to soothe the pain.

- Place ice chips in a clean baby sock and hold it against inflamed gums for 10 to 15 minutes at a time.

Herbalists suggest herb teas for babies that have trouble sleeping, or just to help them be more comfortable. These teas contain chamomile, hops, catnip, and passionflower. Traditional Medicinals brand has a tea containing all of these called "Nighty Night," or Celestial Seasonings chamomile tea with other soothing herbs can be used. NOTE: Teas should be diluted, not full strength, and not given to children under 2 years of age. Some children may have allergies to herbal products. Homeopathic remedies are also used for teething. The main one used is Chamomilla, 6x potency.

Conventional remedies that contain the numbing agent benzocaine, can be used, although such products may contain dyes and artificial sweeteners such as saccharin. You may want to check your health food store to see if there are similar pain relievers that don't contain such unwanted ingredients.

CHAPTER 5

Plaque and Gum Disease

If you're like most people, you probably believe that *plaque* is the "stuff that builds up on your teeth when you don't brush," which leads to cavities (also called caries). In fact, however, plaque is *not* leftover food but a buildup of different types of bacteria and the toxic products they create. Plaque sticks to the tooth surfaces and gum tissue. It is so sticky that once it hardens, it can only be removed in the dentist's office.

Certain types of bacteria in plaque produce tooth decay, while other types cause gum disease. If you want to see these bacteria close up, a dentist with a microscope will show them to you. This is exactly what Antonj van Leeuwenhoek, a Dutch scientist, did about 300 years ago. He had invented the microscope and was looking for things to put under it, so he decided to scrape some plaque from his teeth. When he saw the assorted variety of bacteria and microorganisms he was amazed and called them "animalcules," which means "tiny animals."

In 1965, Dr. Jerome Mittelman wanted to see these for himself, so he mixed a scraping of material from around the tooth with some mouthwash. Then he placed the mixture under a phase microscope, which revealed *live* bacteria in action. Dr. Mittelman says that when the average intelligent patient sees these bacteria swimming around in mouthwash and still creating gum disease, the dentist no longer has to say, "Brush and floss." That patient is on his way to the drugstore to pick up whatever is necessary to get rid of those germs. Dentists who have this microscope will use it periodically to show patients how much progress they have made in getting rid of these unwanted guests.

Our goal in writing this book is to help prevent the growth and multiplication of this army that is so dangerous to your child's dental and overall physical health.

Losing More Than Teeth

Back in 1970, Samuel Charles Miller, D.D.S., professor of periodontia and chief of the Department of Periodontia at New York University Dental School, wrote about the possible relationship of mouth germs to diseases. He thought that these germs could possibly be related to the following diseases:

- *Nervous system:* neuralgia, neuritis, and neurosis
- *Cardiovascular system:* infective endocarditis, rheumatic carditis, myocarditis, and pericarditis
- *Gastrointestinal tract:* gastritis, gastric ulcer, duodenal ulcer, colitis, cholecystitis, and appendicitis
- *Respiratory system:* head colds, chest colds, sinusitis, tonsillitis, chronic bronchitis, asthma, and pulmonary abscess
- *Bony joints:* fibrositis, osteoarthritis, and rheumatoid arthritis
- *Muscles:* myositis
- *Genitourinary tract:* nephritis and pyelitis
- *Skin:* acne vulgaris, furunculosis, herpes simplex, herpes zoster, urticaria, and angioneurotic edema
- *Blood:* anemia, bacteremia, and septicemia
- *Glands:* diabetes mellitus and thyroiditis
- *Ear:* tinnitus, toxic neuritis, and mastoiditis
- *Eye:* iritis, iridocyclitis, conjunctivitis, and keratitis

Not much attention was given to Dr. Miller's suggestions. Today, however, we are seeing more and more evidence that germs from the mouth can and do cause disease. Gastric or peptic ulcers (in the stomach) were always thought to result from eating spicy foods or from stress. Now we know that most of them are caused by bacterial infection. The bacterium *Helicobacter pylori* causes about 90% of stomach ulcers. One of the ways that *H. pylori* gets into the body is through the mouth.

Heart disease is also being linked to mouth bacteria. In an ABC news interview early in 1999, University of Minnesota dentists reported that seemingly harmless bacteria from dental plaque escape from the mouth into the bloodstream and can reach the heart. In animal experiments, they found that within 30 minutes, the bacteria began to produce blood clots, an early stage of heart attack. And the higher the bacteria level, the more irregular the animal's heartbeats became. At the highest bacteria levels the animals died within minutes. The bacteria *Streptococcus sanguis* and *Porphyromonas gingivalis* that caused this destruction are the types that most people have in their mouths, according to University of Minnesota researcher Dr. Mark Herzberg.

Referring to the mouth, Dr. Herzberg said, "It's like having a chronic wound, 9 inches across, exposed to an enormous amount of bacteria which are proving to be very dangerous." The clotting factor found on the surface of the bacteria used in the study (*S. sanguis*) is found in 60% of the same type of bacteria in people. And people with advanced gum disease are 4.5 times more likely to have coronary heart disease.

According to Andrew Weil, M.D., lung diseases such as pneumonia, bronchitis, and emphysema are also present to a greater extent in people with gum disease. Diabetes is another risk associated with gum disease, according to Dr. Weil. Researchers are doing further studies to understand the relationship between gum disease and chronic diseases. The question is, how can you prevent these bacteria from growing in numbers that will overwhelm your immune system and that of your child, allowing invasion of the bacteria into the bloodstream? The answer is within reach—as close as your toothbrush and floss.

How Plaque Causes Decay and Gum Disease

Plaque begins forming on your teeth in as few as 4 hours after brushing. New dental plaque is soft and can easily be removed by brushing and flossing the teeth. So it's important to brush your teeth and that of your child at least twice a day and to floss daily. When it's not removed, however, plaque can lead you down a road to gum disease (gingivitis), periodontal disease, and tooth decay.

When dental plaque is not removed from the tooth surfaces by brushing and flossing, it hardens or mineralizes and is then called *calculus* or *tartar*. Calculus is actually the dead bodies of bacteria that pile up over time and become hard. The old plaque can form above or below the gum line. The bacteria that sticks to calculus can cause gum disease or eventually periodontal disease where the attachment of the tooth to the bone is disrupted. When the plaque has hardened, the tough, crusty deposit can no longer be removed by brushing and flossing. A dental hygienist will have to remove it with special instruments. It is important that this be done without causing injury to the soft gums.

The rate at which plaque forms and where it forms can vary from one person to another. Some people form heavy calculus deposits rapidly, while others form little or none. This has to do with differences in the amount of saliva, the types of plaque bacteria, and dietary factors. Getting a professional cleaning every 6 months, or more frequently as recommended by your dentist, can help reduce the formation of calculus.

Gingivitis

Plaque or calculus (tartar) buildup along the gum line can inflame the gums. This inflammation of the gum tissue is called *gingivitis* (gingiva is another name for the gums). The gums may be sore, bleed easily and appear puffy, soft and swollen. The gum color may be reddish or purple. At this stage of gum disease, the bony structures around the teeth are still intact. Blood on the toothbrush or dental floss is one of the earliest and most common signs of gingivitis. Your gums and those of your child should never bleed while brushing or flossing. It's important to keep up the brushing and flossing because during early stages of gingivitis, there may be no symptoms.

The good news about gingivitis is that it is preventable and reversible through good brushing and flossing techniques and a good diet and supplements. On the other hand, if oral hygiene habits and diet are poor, gingivitis may progress and become long-lasting or chronic.

Chronic gingivitis is common in children. According to the American Academy of Periodontology, 97% of school-aged children will get gingivitis. A child may have gingival inflammation without detectable loss of bone or tooth attachments, and it will usually get better after a thorough removal of bacterial deposits and improved daily oral hygiene practices (brushing and flossing). When gingivitis is neglected, it will eventually progress to periodontal disease.

Gingivitis is more prevalent among children with diabetes or asthma.

Periodontal Disease

Periodontal disease affects the periodontium (the supporting structures of the teeth). It can be so severe that the teeth loosen and fall out. Teeth sit in sockets in the bones of the upper and lower jaws in *alveolar* (hollow) bone, which does not hold the teeth in place. The teeth are actually held in place by connective tissue called *periodontal ligaments* that extend from the roots of the teeth into the sockets and anchor the teeth.

Bacteria in plaque play a major role in periodontal disease. When there is continued irritation from the plaque, the collar of gum tissue (the sulcus) around the bone will widen and pull away from the tooth. This makes more room for the bacteria, and the supporting structures begin to break down.

As a result, the part of the bone that supports the teeth or the ligaments that hold the teeth securely in place become inflamed and are eventually destroyed. Pockets around the teeth enlarge and deepen, and more potent forms of bacteria take up residence in these pockets. Eventually, there is so much ligament and bone loss that the tooth is not anchored in the socket and will loosen. The pressures from chewing will make the tooth even looser, and it will fall out or need to be extracted. This disease process is generally not reversible and will require treatment from a dental professional specializing in periodontal disease.

You can see the importance of starting early to keep your child's mouth clean and healthy. By doing this, your child will develop good oral hygiene habits that will protect his or her health. Your child's mouth is connected to the rest of his body. Healthy teeth are a legacy that will do more for your child in his or her lifetime than all the riches money can buy.

According to the American Academy of Pediatric Dentistry (AAPD), for many decades, periodontal conditions in young children were mostly ignored. Now dentists realize that periodontal disease starts early, and they are starting to do something about it. Recent studies show that almost 40% of children in the 24-to-36-month age group have at least mild inflammation of the gums. Periodontitis in children and preadolescents, conditions that progress rapidly and result in the loss of primary and permanent teeth, are increasing in frequency. Up to 9% of 5 to 11 year olds and up to 46% of 12 to 15 year olds have gum disease. The AAPD now recommends that parents and dentists put greater emphasis on the prevention, early diagnosis, and treatment of gingival and periodontal disease in children.

Warning Signs of Periodontal Disease

- Gums that bleed when you or your child brush or floss
- Gums that are red, swollen, or tender
- Gums that have pulled away from teeth (recession), sometimes exposing roots
- Infection including purulence (pus) between the teeth and gums when the gums are pressed
- Permanent teeth that are loose or separating
- Any changes in the way teeth fit together when you bite
- Bad breath not improved by brushing and flossing

Note: Calculus and plaque may not be visible to the naked eye, and gum disease may not be painful. Only your dentist can detect these problems, so your child needs regular checkups to catch these problems in the early stages.

Fighting Plaque

If periodontal disease is present, the usual treatment is called *scaling*. Scaling and root planing are nonsurgical techniques that remove plaque and tartar from below the gum line. Tooth root surfaces are cleaned and smoothed with specially designed instruments. This treatment should restore the health of the gums. However, the gums may have receded, exposing the roots of the teeth. This is due to the irreversible bone loss as a result of the previous periodontal disease. This can lead to tooth sensitivity.

Is removing plaque the only way to have healthy gums and teeth? Dr. E. Cheraskin, who is both an M.D. and a dentist, has proven that there is another side to the story. Dr. Cheraskin gave a supplement containing 500 milligrams of vitamin C to young boys for 90 days and then checked the health of their teeth and gums. He found that no matter how poorly or how well the boys brushed their teeth, those that took the vitamin C had a cleaner mouth! In another study, he found that just brushing the teeth without use of vitamin C resulted in a 30% improvement in gum disease (gingivitis). However, even in people who did not brush their teeth, and just took vitamin C, there was a 45% reduction in gingivitis. Adding brushing and vitamin C together gave a 58% improvement in gingivitis. Is it just a coincidence that the classical signs of vitamin C deficiency (scurvy) include severe gingivitis, bleeding gums, and loosening of teeth due to the loss of the supporting connective tissue? It is obvious that gum tissue is healthier in the presence of vitamin C. Dr. Linus Pauling, a two-time Nobel Prize winner, pointed out that gum disease is a form of scurvy. This means that vitamin C intake is too low in people who have gum disease.

Breast milk can supply your infant with vitamin C if you have a good supply of the vitamin in your diet. Multivitamin drops that contain vitamin C are also available for infants and very young children. For older children, chewable multivitamins or vitamin C tablets can help keep gums healthy and teeth clean. Make sure that chewable vitamins don't contain sugar, and give them with meals so that the after-eating brushing will remove any sweetener they may contain.

Another vitamin important for gum health is the B vitamin folic acid. The gums and all the surface tissues in the mouth use large amounts of folic acid to stay healthy. This B vitamin is found in fresh green leafy vegetables and brewer's yeast. If these foods are not part of your child's diet, look for folic acid in the liquid or chewable vitamins. There should be at least 200 micrograms (a day) of folic acid; 400 micrograms is better. Folic acid is also important for cell growth throughout the body and for keeping the heart and blood vessels healthy.

CHAPTER 6

A Plan for Baby's Teeth

It's never too early to start infant oral health care. Ideally, this care begins with health counseling for parents-to-be. Your dentist can provide guidance including preventive education, so you will be ready to take the steps to give your baby a lifetime of freedom from oral disease.

According to the American Academy of Pediatric Dentistry (AAPD), the most effective time to begin a preventive program for your baby is during the prenatal period—before he or she is born. The AAPD and other dental and parent advocacy organizations now recommend that preventive dentistry information be given in all prenatal classes.

Once your baby cuts his or her first tooth, the first dental visit should occur within 6 months and no later than 12 months of age, according to the American Dental Association (ADA). In any case, as soon as the first tooth comes in, parents should begin brushing the tooth. Oral health, however, will begin before that (see below). At the visit, your dentist should take a thorough medical and dental history and do a thorough oral examination. We will discuss your child's first and subsequent dental visits in detail in a later chapter.

Your dentist can determine the likelihood of the child's developing dental disease and will set a timing schedule for checkups. Topics the dentist may discuss include how the teeth will develop, feeding practices, oral habits such as thumb sucking and pacifiers, injury prevention (play objects, pacifiers, car seats), oral hygiene, and effects of diet on the teeth. Dentists who perform such services for infants should be prepared to provide therapy when needed or should refer the family to a health professional trained properly for the necessary treatment.

According to the AAPD, "The infant oral health care visit should be seen as the foundation on which a lifetime of preventive education and dental care can be built, in order to help assure optimal oral health into childhood."

A way to reduce gum disease that you may not have known about is to have your child stay away from cigarette smoke. Even secondhand smoke, according to Andrew Weil, M.D., can increase the risk of developing gum disease. This may be a result of the fact that cigarette smoke constricts blood vessels and reduces the blood flow to the gums. We recommend the antioxidant nutrient coenzyme Q_{10} (CoQ_{10}), which is very healthy for the gums. It is now found in some natural-ingredient toothpastes.

Caring for Gums and Tiny Teeth

Before your baby or young toddler goes off to sleep, you should do more than kiss him or her goodnight. Be sure you are caring for your child's tiny teeth—and even before they arrive, for his or her gums. Many dentists advise parents to start dental care within the first few days after their child's birth by gently wiping their baby's gums with a moist washcloth after each feeding. Establishing this pattern early on will help the child accept a brush once the first teeth begin to appear.

When you wipe your baby's teeth, a better choice for the "toothbrush" is a damp sterile gauze pad. If you use a washcloth it should be very clean, and a fresh one should be used each time. You wouldn't want to put germs in your baby's mouth. Besides ensuring that your baby has a clean, sweet mouth, this massaging of the gums is also good for blood circulation that promotes healthy gums.

Two sets of teeth normally develop: the *primary dentition* or "baby" teeth, and the *secondary dentition* or permanent teeth. The first tooth "buds" start to grow when the fetus is 10 weeks old and tooth development continues throughout pregnancy. The tooth buds are under the gums at birth.

As soon as the first tooth appears, begin using a small, soft-bristled toothbrush to clean the tooth after nursing or eating. Don't cover the brush with toothpaste. Young children tend to swallow most of the toothpaste, and swallowing too much fluoridated toothpaste can cause permanent spots on their teeth, called *dental fluorosis*. However, as you will see in a later chapter, this is just the tip of the iceberg of the many problems with fluoride.

An alternative to a toothbrush is a finger toothbrush and gum massager. This finger-shaped cap goes over your finger. It has a small soft brush on it. It's less frightening to a baby than a brush and can be used to massage gums sore from teething. It can also be sterilized in boiling water or frozen like a teething ring. Called the Infa-Dent®, it is available from Laclede, Inc. (see Resources). During the massage, include pleasant "baby talk" to help prepare your baby psychologically to enjoy the cleaning experience.

Baby's First Teeth: Tooth Eruption Patterns

Usually the first baby teeth to come into the mouth are the 2 bottom front teeth. They begin to appear when your child is about 6 to 8 months old. The 4 upper front teeth follow them. The remainder of your baby's teeth will appear periodically, usually in pairs on each side of the jaw, until the child is about 2½ years old.

By the time your child is 2½ years old, all 20 baby teeth will most likely have come in. From this point until the child is 5 to 6 years of age, his or her first permanent teeth will begin to erupt. Some of the permanent teeth replace baby teeth; others don't. Do not worry if some teeth are a few months early or late. Every child is different.

We know that to have healthy teeth and gums, there must be daily plaque removal from all surfaces of the tooth through brushing and interdental cleaning. Interdental cleaning means using a small "proxy" brush to get in between the teeth. What do healthy gums look like? Healthy gums have the following features:

- Pink or coral pink color (normal variations in color depend on race and complexion)
- Firm, resilient tissues
- "Orange-peel" texture (known as stippling)
- Shape that follows the contour of the teeth and forms a scalloped edge
- No areas of redness, swelling, or inflammation
- No bleeding during daily plaque removal

Even though baby teeth will eventually be lost, they are just as important as the adult teeth. They not only hold the space for incoming permanent teeth, but are also important for biting and chewing food, speech, and physical appearance. Early tooth loss due to dental decay can have a serious impact on your child's self-esteem and confidence in his or her appearance. A complete set of healthy primary teeth allows proper development of a child's jaw and face. For this reason, it is important to teach your child from an early age the importance of eating a healthy diet and practicing daily oral hygiene to maintain healthy teeth and gums for a lifetime of smiles.

Children exposed to tobacco smoke from parents' cigarettes may have delays in formation of permanent teeth, say researchers reporting in a recent issue of the *Journal of Clinical Pediatric Dentistry.* Exposing a child to tobacco smoke can delay tooth development by an average of 4 months. The most significant delays were seen when both parents smoked.

Teething Trouble

We talked about teething problems in chapter 4. Here are some more helpful ideas to get your baby through this stressful time. Teething may make your baby restless and irritable. However, all your baby's problems may not be related to teething. If fever, vomiting, or diarrhea occurs don't automatically think it's teething, as it is not generally the cause of these conditions. See your doctor first.

Here are some signs that your baby may be teething:

- Red cheeks or rash on cheeks
- Increased saliva or drooling
- Restlessness
- Irritability
- Loss of appetite

What to do? Let your child chew on a cold, hard object, such as a frozen teething ring. The coldness helps ease the discomfort, and the hardness will speed up the eruption of the tooth. Massaging your child's gums with a clean finger can help reduce pain and discomfort during teething. There are teething gels or ointments (ask your pharmacist or health store person for a brand name) that are used to numb the gums and reduce the discomfort. Try to use products that don't contain artificial colors, artificial sweeteners, or sugar. Teething cookies or biscuits are not a good choice as they contain sugar and may lead to tooth decay.

Clove oil *(Syzygium aromaticum)* is a natural anesthetic that reduces inflammation. It may be used for teething. Never put it on full strength. It should always be diluted because the full-strength oil will cause blistering. You can mix one drop of clove oil with 1 to 2 tablespoons of canola or olive oil and rub it on sore gums.

Motivating Children to Clean Their Teeth Properly

At around 18 months of age your child will usually be eager to mimic the things you do, including tooth brushing. You can set a good example by taking care of your own dental hygiene. Dr. A. J. Chialastri D.D.S., director of Pediatric Dental Medicine at St. Christopher's Hospital for Children in Phildelphia warns that although toddlers may want to brush their teeth, most of them don't have enough hand coordination to do it properly until about age 5 (6 or 7 according to the ADA). He suggests that either Mom or Dad supervise and follow up with a more thorough cleansing until children reach an age when they have the ability to brush their teeth properly.

Dr. Chialastri trys to make the dental cleaning process fun. Here are some of his tips for parents to make mouth care more pleasant for your child:

- Wean babies off the baby bottle by 12 to 14 months of age.
- Choose a children's toothpaste with a mild flavor and use a child-size soft-bristled toothbrush decorated with a favorite cartoon character or color.
- Make brushing teeth a game by letting your child brush your teeth before you brush the child's.
- Teach your child proper brushing techniques. Move the tooth-brush in small circles on both the inside and the outside of each tooth, making sure to reach the gum line, where cavity-causing plaque tends to collect. Then use a back-and-forth motion to clean the biting surface of the teeth.
- Encourage your child to establish a daily pattern for brushing their teeth. It is recommended to brush teeth in the morning and at night and right after every meal. (This may not always be possible. See below for an alternative plan.)
- Don't begin flossing your child's teeth until they begin to touch each other, usually around age 4 or 5. At that age flossing is recommended every night. (See below for more tips on floss-ing.)

Brushing Tips

Tooth brushing will remove dental plaque and other debris from your child's teeth. Plaque, as we have noted, plays a primary role in oral disease such as tooth decay and gum disease. The best way to remove plaque from the tooth surface on a daily home care basis is through tooth brushing and some form of between-the-teeth clean-ing.

The following toothbrush technique is commonly recommended by dental hygienists. You should see your dental hygienist to make sure that you are using the best technique.

1. Use a soft-bristled brush (synthetic bristles are preferred be-cause natural bristles tend to harbor oral bacteria, as the bris-

tles are more porous). Be sure it is the right size (generally smaller is better than larger).

2. Place the bristles at a 45-degree angle to the teeth. Slide the tips of the brush under the gums.
3. Jiggle the bristles very gently so that any plaque growing under the gum will be removed.
4. Be sure to brush the outside, the tongue side, and the chewing surfaces of your child's teeth.
5. For the front teeth, brush the inside surfaces of the upper and lower jaws by tilting the brush vertically and making several up-and-down strokes with the front part of the brush over the teeth and gum tissues.
6. Change the brush's position with each tooth.
7. Brushing your child's tongue will help freshen his or her breath. Debris and bacteria can collect on the tongue and cause bad breath.

To prevent plaque damage, be sure to brush your child's teeth at least once every day, preferably at bedtime. Adding a brush time after breakfast increases your chances of thorough daily plaque removal.

What about brushing before bed? This is the important one. If you have to miss a brushing, the bedtime one is probably the worst one to miss. If you don't get rid of the bacteria and sugar that cause cavities, they have all night to do harm. While you and your child are awake, saliva helps keep the mouth clean. When you are asleep, there is less saliva produced to clean the mouth. For this reason it is important to brush before bedtime.

Don't rush to brush. A thorough brushing should take at least 3 minutes. Brushing the teeth too vigorously or using a hard-bristled toothbrush causes the gums to recede and exposes root surfaces. It also wears down the tooth structure. Both of these conditions can lead to tooth sensitivity.

Again, a pea-sized amount of toothpaste is all you need, should you choose to use toothpaste. Replace toothbrushes when the bristles begin to spread. Some toothbrushes have a color indicator that lets you know when to change to a new one. A worn-out toothbrush will not properly clean your teeth. A study that was published in the *Journal of Dental Research* showed that compared to a 3-month worn toothbrush, a new brush removed 30.7% more plaque.

> The toothbrush was invented by an enterprising English prisoner named William Addis about 1770. He started by using rags, but then got the idea of boring holes in the end of a small bone and gluing tufted bristles into them. When he was released from prison, he became a successful toothbrush manufacturer.

When brushing your child's teeth you may find that you have problems. Children tend to wiggle and squirm and get into awkward positions. Here are some things you can try for children up to 2 or 3 years old:

- Have your child lie on the bed and put his or her head on a pillow, then sit next to your child so you are face to face. Or put your child face up on your lap on a pillow. This position makes brushing a caring, nurturing time. Both positions will properly support your child's head and give you the needed control to effectively brush.
- If your child is standing, have his or her back to you with the head tilted slightly and resting against your body. This will give your child better balance during the brushing.
- Your child may like to hold a mirror while you brush and floss the teeth so he or she can see what is being done.
- Make a game of tongue brushing, asking your child to stick out his or her tongue as far as possible. You only need to brush the front third or half of the tongue. Going further back may gag the child.

Toothbrushes are available for all age groups and come in various shapes, sizes, softness, and colors. Some toothbrushes are specifically designed for children's small mouths and hands. Children will usually have better control of large-handled brushes. Be certain the brush you select has soft nylon bristles and is small enough to maneuver inside your child's mouth.

The following tips will help you make certain your child is getting the most out of his or her toothbrush:

- Clean toothbrushes thoroughly after use and dry in an open place. Consider storing toothbrushes in the bedroom where there may be less chance of contamination.
- If several toothbrushes are stored in the same place, allow brushes to dry without touching each other or surfaces dampened by other toothbrushes.
- Normal wear can bend the bristles and move them out of line. Splayed bristles lose their ability to properly remove plaque from teeth. When the bristles become bent or frayed, a new brush is needed.
- As a simple rule of thumb, toothbrushes should be changed every 3 months, or more often if the bristles show wear and tear. Also change the brush after an illness or when the bristles begin to stiffen.

What About Electric Toothbrushes and Water Irrigators?

Although electric toothbrushes are good cleaning aids, we don't recommend them for children. These brushes, such as the Rota-Dent (see Resources) do a good job of removing plaque and reducing inflammation. However, just as with regular toothbrushes, little hands are not coordinated enough to use such devices. They should not be left where children can get them. The same is true for water irrigators. Using water, by the way, is not a substitute for flossing. After floss loosens the plaque, water is useful in washing it away so that the free plaque doesn't sit between the teeth. Again, don't allow young children to use these devices unsupervised.

How to Floss

Flossing helps to remove plaque from in between your teeth, in areas that your toothbrush can't reach. Dr. C.C. Bass, dean of Tulane Medical School in Louisiana, discovered the importance of flossing back in the 1940s. After retiring as dean, Dr. Bass devoted himself to studying tooth decay. He found that as long as the germs that cause tooth decay were exposed to saliva, they couldn't do their damaging job. Once plaque formed, saliva couldn't get through this shield that protected the germs. However, refined sugars went right through—immediately. Germs use this sugar to break down the teeth. So even brushing right after a meal could be too late to protect the teeth if sugars got in under the plaque. The best protection is to keep this plaque shield from forming. Since toothbrush bristles can't get in between the teeth, flossing is very important.

Effective flossing removes the colonies of germs and disorganizes them before they start to form hard plaque. So flossing is not just for removing food from between the teeth. Dr. Bass found that flossing once a day was enough to keep the plaque from hardening.

It is really not the space between the teeth you are flossing, but the tooth surface. Start flossing your child's teeth when the teeth touch each other and you can no longer brush in between them. You will have to floss your child's teeth until he or she is capable of doing it.

Don't be discouraged with your first attempt at flossing your child's teeth. Flossing (whether it is for yourself or your child) is a skill that is learned. It takes practice. After a while, it will take only a few minutes of your time. You may want to see your dental hygienist for a demonstration. Here is some advice on how to floss:

1. Wrap about 18 inches of floss around the middle fingers of your hands.
2. Holding the floss tightly (use your thumbs and forefingers) gently guide the floss between your child's teeth. Never "snap" the floss, as this can cut the gums.
3. When the floss reaches the gum line, curve it into a C-shape against one tooth and gently slide it into the space between the gum and the tooth putting pressure against the tooth.
4. Gently scrape the side of the tooth with the floss.
5. Move to a clean area of floss after doing one or two teeth.
6. Repeat this method on all your child's teeth.

If you do not have good finger dexterity, you may find it helpful to use a commercial floss holder. However, this is a "last resort" since you can't floss really effectively with a floss holder. Or, to make the flossing job easier, you may want to tie the ends of the floss together in a circle instead of using just one long piece of floss. Then hold the floss tightly between the thumbs and forefingers to floss. This circle method will be easier for your child to use once he or she is ready to floss solo. You may need to help your child floss his or her back teeth, which are the hardest to reach and which collect the most cavity-causing residue. Remember to be gentle when inserting floss between your child's teeth and under the gum line. Flossing can injure the gums if done improperly. The gums may bleed and be sore for the first few days that you floss, but they should heal and the bleeding should stop once all the bacteria are removed. Gums that are sore can be rinsed with warm salt water (just a pinch of salt in a glass of water) or warm chamomile tea (very soothing).

Establish a regular pattern and time for flossing, so that you don't miss any of your child's teeth. Move from one side of the upper mouth to the other and then do the bottom teeth, for example. Note that most children cannot floss their own teeth properly until about the age of 10.

Which floss should you use? The purpose of floss is to cut through, disorganize, and remove plaque from areas in between the teeth where most gum disease and cavities start. To do this job the floss should splay out (separate), becoming numerous cutting edges that actually slice off the plaque. Waxed floss cannot do this. The wax keeps the filaments (strands) of the floss stuck together. Originally, floss was waxed in order to prevent it from becoming entangled in the container. And, of course, people liked the waxed floss, because it seemed to slip in between the teeth more easily.

But does waxed floss disorganize plaque and remove it? It may push it around some, but unless the floss separates, it's really not effective. Some floss is labeled "unwaxed." However, it has a starchy filler binding it, so that it cannot splay out. Holding it under warm water will wash out the filler.

One company that makes an unwaxed floss is Butler GUM (see Resources) called "Right Kind" dental floss. This may have the starchy binder, but it can be removed as noted above. The POH (Personal Oral Hygiene) company (see Resources) makes another very good unwaxed floss.

The American Academy of Pediatric Dentistry and Oral-B Laboratories surveyed parents about their concerns regarding the oral health of their children. According to the survey, almost 25% of parents expressed concern about proper brushing and flossing techniques. About 33% were concerned about cavities, and the third largest concern was for the maintenance of healthy teeth and gums for their children. One of the recommendations based on the survey was that oral care patterns for children can be easily established if the behaviors are taught in stages that correspond to the child's development: an "ages and stages" approach.

Toothpastes and Mouthwashes: Which Ones Are Best?

Toothpaste has been around for a long time. The ancient healer Hippocrates had recipes for making toothpaste in 377 B.C. Manufacturers add many substances to toothpaste in the hope of reducing plaque and keeping teeth and gums healthy. Some ingredients should be included in toothpastes (and mouthwashes) and other things should not be there. Some of the ingredients are there to prevent the toothpaste from being stringy or hardening or are added for taste. Other ingredients are said to prevent caries, tartar (plaque), and gum disease; desensitize or whiten teeth; and prevent bad breath. There are abrasives and foaming agents, moisturizing agents, binders/thickeners, and sweeteners.

If it sounds like a chemistry lesson, you're right—and many of these ingredients are not good for tiny teeth and delicate gums (or anyone's mouth for that matter!). Here are some of the ingredients you wouldn't want to put into your child's mouth:

Abrasives: These include silica, calcium carbonate, dicalcium phosphate, and alumina (which contains aluminum, a metal linked to Alzheimer's disease). According to Dr. Jerome Mittelman, "Americans daily brush their teeth with stones, animal bones, and sand particles without being aware of it." Calcium carbonate comes from stones, dicalcium phosphate is bone, and the silica used in most toothpastes comes from sand. These abrasives damage tooth enamel. There is a natural source of silica, however, called the horsetail plant. This type of silica is much less abrasive and will not harm the teeth.

Brushing for years with abrasive-containing toothpastes in an attempt to whiten teeth will have the opposite effect: wearing down the enamel exposes the dentin below, which is a yellowish color. Even some "natural" toothpastes sold in health stores contain these abrasives.

Sodium lauryl sulfate: According to TV medical doctor, Dean Edell, this common detergent is found in many toothpastes. Research shows that it dries out the protective mucous layer lining the mouth, leaving it vulnerable to irritants (such as acidic foods) and to bacteria. Researchers found that using toothpaste without sodium lauryl sulfate can help people who have chronic canker sores.

Pyrophosphate compounds: Researchers at the University of Maryland School of Dentistry found that pyrophosphate compounds, found in so-called tartar-control toothpastes, can irritate sensitive skin in allergy-prone people. If you or your child have burning, itching, or red cracked skin around the mouth, check your toothpaste for this ingredient.

Artificial flavors, sweeteners, and dyes: Artificial flavors—and dyes especially—cause allergies or can produce toxic reactions in many children. A baby or child's immature liver cannot do the detoxifying job that an adult liver can do. This puts a burden on the baby's liver and also on the immune system if allergies result. Artificial sweeteners can cause problems as well. Saccharin has been caught in the "Does it or doesn't it cause cancer" debate for many years. It can be absorbed through the gums. It is rated as carcinogenic by the International Agency for Research on Cancer. Saccharin may also cause a woman's delicate reproductive cycle to become disrupted. Sorbitol can cause diarrhea in some individuals. Aspartame is another substance that babies are not equipped to process with their immature liver and kidneys. Polysorbate 80 may be contaminated with 1,4 dioxane, which is found in pesticides and paints and is a health hazard if inhaled, absorbed through the skin (or gums), or eaten. It can cause drowsiness, headaches, nausea, vomiting, and irritation to the eyes, nose, throat, and skin, according to the National Safety Council Environmental Health Center.

FD&C Blue No. 1, a coal-tar dye often found in toothpaste, causes cancer in animals.

Triclosan: This chemical agent is an antimicrobial. It is a disinfectant usually found in antibacterial soaps.

> Popeye was right. Leafy green vegetables are good sources of vitamin K, which can prevent tooth decay by counteracting acid formation by mouth bacteria. It works as well or better than fluoride. This amazing vitamin is also essential to the formation of osteocalcin, a protein that attracts calcium and helps build it into bone, including the teeth.

We will discuss fluoride and the dangers to your child that this toxic substance represents in a later chapter. We have provided information on fluoride for parents who choose to give it to their children, but we don't recommend that fluoride be given in *any* form—not in toothpaste, drinking water, or in tooth sealants.

For dentists who do recommend the use of fluoride-containing toothpaste, recent research shows that brushing should be done with a pea-sized amount of fluoride-containing toothpaste. This amount gives children just enough for cavity protection, and also decreases the risk of *fluorosis,* a damaging condition caused by overingestion of fluoride which usually shows up as white flecks on the tooth enamel.

> TV doctor Dean Edel says, "Kids are getting too much fluoride in toothpaste." He goes on to say that the first thing that too much fluoride will do is stain the teeth (fluorosis). "We're seeing more fluorosis, and the reason is that your kid is getting too much of it," says Dr. Dean. He found that children who used fluoride toothpaste before age 6 had almost twice the rate of fluorosis as children not exposed at that age.

Toothpaste with Whiteners

Not everyone is born with white teeth. Tooth color is actually inherited, like eye and hair color. There is a range of colors from white to yellow. The best way to keep teeth looking their brightest is to clean them well. Trying to whiten teeth artificially can actually worsen the problem. When the tooth enamel is weakened, as it does when teeth are bleached, the tooth becomes more sensitive to temperature changes. Artificial whitening defeats the purpose. Whitened teeth absorb stains more easily, requiring repeated bleaching. Don't start this "merry-go-round" of whitening.

> In a recent survey at an American Dental Association meeting, 88% of the dentists said that the number of tooth-whitening procedures they perform has increased in the last 3 years. Fifty-two percent of these dentists also reported an increase in tooth hypersensitivity.

Are tooth whiteners safe? The main ingredient in whiteners is hydrogen peroxide—in higher strengths than the solution used for cleaning cuts. Dr. Clifford W. Whall, Jr., director of product evaluation at the ADA, and others say that whitening, if not done properly, can kill gum tissue or damage the teeth.

Animal studies suggest that high concentrations of hydrogen peroxide can cause irreversible cell damage and may enhance some cancer-causing substances. Combination whitener and toothpaste preparations contain less peroxide but are recommended for use twice a day, presumably for life. So the damage will be there, only it will develop more slowly.

In an article in the *Journal of the American Dental Association,* Dr. Chakway Siew, who heads the ADA Research Institute's Department of Toxicology, had this to say about the active chemical agents in whiteners: "[They] ultimately break down to hydrogen peroxide and release oxygen free radicals, a very active species." Free radicals are reactive chemicals that can destroy cells in the body. These free radicals can harm gum tissue and delay wound healing. Your body uses up vitamin C and other antioxidants to inactivate these free radicals. Since vitamin C is so important for healthy gums, any process that uses it up is not good for mouth health. The effect of lifetime exposure to low-level hydrogen peroxide is unknown, the experts say.

Good Toothpaste Ingredients

For babies and very young children we recommend toothpaste that is as natural as possible and fluoride-free. Because babies and young children will swallow whatever is put in their mouths, the sensible thing to do would be to have a toothpaste that was ingestible—one that they *could* eat with no problems. And there are such toothpastes. One that contains the enzymes found in mother's milk, lactoferrin and lactoperoxidase, can reduce the bacteria that cause gum and tooth disease (First Teeth, Laclede Professional Products, Inc.; see Resources). It doesn't contain saccharin, fluoride, or harmful preservatives and is naturally flavored.

We also recommend tooth-cleaning products made with Peelu. Peelu is a tree that is well known throughout Asia, the Middle East, and parts of Africa. In Islamic countries it is called Meswak. The botanical name is *Salvadora persica*. It is also known as the "toothbrush tree." The branches of this tree have been used for centuries for tooth cleaning, disinfecting the mouth, and refreshing the breath. These branches are ground into a powder, and a nonabrasive toothpaste is made from the plant fibers. Experiments done in Saudi Arabia and in the Department of Chemistry, Indiana University, Bloomington, Indiana, show that Peelu contains antibacterial substances and is an anti-inflammatory. In India and Persia it is one of the oldest means of tooth brightening.

As mentioned above, Dr. Andrew Weil recommends CoQ_{10} for healthy gums. Some of the natural toothpastes are adding this ingredient.

Mouthwash: Does It Work?

Some ads for antiseptic mouthwashes would have us believe that their products kill germs. Most mouthwashes are simply breath fresheners and do not eliminate bacteria.

Adding zinc, aloe, or grapefruit seed extracts to toothpaste may protect against viral and bacterial infections of the mouth. While some toothpastes and mouth rinses may kill bacteria in the mouth, most are useless against viruses.

According to the FDA's Advisory Review Panel on Over-the-Counter Oral Health Care Products, the belief that regular use of mouthwash will prevent gum disease is an "absurd notion," and is "based upon tradition, promotional appeal by manufacturers and misunderstandings." Also, mouthwashes may increase the time for mouth wounds and sores to heal because they contain alcohol or chemicals that irritate tissue. By killing beneficial organisms, mouthwashes may upset the natural balance of organisms that live in the mouth. The panel also said that "bad breath" is not a disease. Although some mouthwashes may kill some germs, this is only temporary. The germs return in about a half hour, according to John Carr, an FDA dentist who worked with the panel. Just as effective and far less dangerous ways to get rid of bad breath are rinsing with water, brushing and flossing, or just eating breakfast, according to the panel.

Alcohol in Mouthwashes

According to the American Academy of Pediatric Dentistry, the ingestion of alcohol-containing mouthwashes presents an avoidable health hazard to infants and young children. Yes, they will drink mouthwash. The Academy emphatically supports efforts to have childproof caps put on these products. They also believe that labels should tell consumers that children under 6 years should not use the products. Use of alcohol-containing mouth rinses by children should be allowed only if specifically recommended by a dentist or physician, and children should be under close adult supervision when using these products.

Alcohol can also dry the mouth and interfere with the production of saliva, our first defense against mouth bacteria. Some mouthwashes can contain up to 70% alcohol—and a young child mistaking mouthwash for soda or iced tea may go into a coma after drinking it.

Mouthwashes That Do No Harm

Do we really need to give our children mouthwashes that contain harsh and possibly harmful ingredients? Cranberry juice may be a better bet. It prevents bladder infections by preventing bacteria from sticking to the bladder walls, and may also prevent bacteria in the mouth from sticking to each other and forming plaque. Cranberries contain an antioxidant, polyphenol, that prevents bacteria from joining together to form plaque on the teeth. But cranberry juice cocktail should not be used, because it contains the sugars fructose and dextrose, which may promote plaque formation.

What are good ingredients that won't harm your child? Here are some: glycerin, aloe vera juice, witch hazel (nonalcoholic), spearmint oil, menthol, and vitamin C. We don't as a rule recommend mouthwashes, but we feel that the Natural Dentist Herbal Mouth and Gum Therapy Daily Oral Rinse for Children and Adults is safe for children. It's sweetened with glycerin and herbs and contains natural flavorings. (See Resources.) There are some herbs that can be used to soothe and help heal gum tissues. Calendula flower and chamomile tea (strained) can also be used as a mouthwash.

One of the authors had a personal experience with chamomile. As a child of 10 or 11 Jean developed stomatitis, an inflammation of the mouth that was very painful. Surprisingly, her pediatrician recommended warm rinses of chamomile tea, which worked very well. Chamomile is a good source of vitamin C and B vitamins, all important nutrients for the gums. It is very soothing on sore gums.

You can make your own antibacterial mouth rinse by mixing 1 cup of warm water, a quarter teaspoon of salt, and a half teaspoon (or the contents of one capsule) of goldenseal powder.

Now that we know how to keep teeth clean, we need to know more about keeping them healthy with good nutrition. The big question to talk about next is, "Should your child eat sweets?"

CHAPTER 7

Sugar and Other Sweet Dangers

More Than Just Teeth Are at Stake

If you love your child, you will prevent him or her from eating too much sugar. Everyone knows that overconsumption of sugar is associated with tooth decay. However, according to scientific research, sugar's health effects reach well beyond the teeth. Sugar in the diet, whether it's obvious like candy or hidden in foods, will hurt your child's health in many other ways. Sugar, especially refined sugar, causes a loss of calcium from the body. This means that the bones as well as the teeth are at risk. Growing children need optimal amounts of calcium for bone growth. Loss of calcium also affects teeth. One of the important mechanisms that protect teeth from the acids that bacteria make requires calcium. In the presence of acid, the enamel of the tooth releases calcium and phosphate, which work together to neutralize the acid. If calcium levels are low because of excess sugar, this protection doesn't work well.

Although tooth enamel is in danger from excess sugar, so are other major systems in your child's body. Sugar in excess depresses the immune system. A decrease in the germ-killing and cancer-prevention ability of immune cells (called natural killer cells) can actually be measured for up to 3 hours after eating sugar. This weakness in immunity affects the ability of the body to fight tooth-decay-causing bacteria and slows the repair of gum tissue. It impairs the body's ability to fight periodontal disease as well. It also affects your child's ability to fight off colds, the flu, and other infections. Cancer cells arise in our bodies every day; a strong immune system (with healthy natural killer cells) is our protection against these cells living long enough to take hold and cause cancer. A sugar-weakened immune system can't fight cancer.

High sugar levels cause changes in our blood-sugar-controlling organ, the pancreas. In children, the pancreas releases small amounts of insulin, the hormone that keeps blood sugar levels normal. Only small amounts are needed even if the child eats lots of sugar and carbohydrates. This is because a child's cells are extremely sensitive to insulin. Cells have to take up insulin in order to regulate blood sugar. Insulin "tells" the cells that there is too much sugar in the blood and the cells won't release more sugar. But eating a lot of sugar has a price tag. Eventually the child's cells lose sensitivity to insulin—a condition known as insulin resistance. Although there are high levels of insulin in the blood, it doesn't work because the cells are resistant to insulin's message. This leads to diabetes and all the diseases that follow: high cholesterol, high blood pressure, and heart disease. Sugar eating helps lay the foundation for these diseases that will show up later in life. So there is a lot more than just your child's teeth at stake.

Sugar Comes in Many Forms

There's a saying: "A rose is a rose" (Gertrude Stein). And sugar, whatever the name, is still sugar. There are many names and not knowing them may make you think that there is less sugar in a food than there really is. If you learn to decipher the various names for sugar that appear on food labels, you can make better choices about what your child eats.

Sugars are carbohydrates. Carbohydrates, which include sugars and starches, are the body's primary source of fuel for energy. Sugars are *simple carbohydrates,* while starches are *complex carbohydrates.* Though both types are broken down in the body to glucose, foods that are high in complex carbohydrates, such as grains and vegetables, usually supply a healthy bonus of vitamins, minerals, and fiber along with the carbohydrates. However, simple carbohydrates from candy, cake, table sugar, syrups, sweetened cereals, and other sources of concentrated sugar contribute "empty calories" that can provide energy, but none of the healthy nutrients found in complex carbohydrates.

Sucrose (table sugar) is just one form of sugar. Food ingredients ending in -ose such as sucrose are sugars. Many foods contain sugars such as high-fructose corn syrup, dextrose, maltose, corn syrup or corn sweetener, and honey which contains glucose. Milk contains lactose. Fruits contain glucose and fructose. There are also sugar "alcohols" (ending in -ol) such as sorbitol, mannitol, xylitol, and maltitol and products made from the alcohols such as isomalt and hydrogenated starch hydrolysates. They are also called polyols. These are found in "sugar-free" candies, cookies, and chewing gums. Sugar alcohols occur naturally in many fruits and vegetables, but are produced commercially from other carbohydrates such as sucrose, glucose, and starch. Other types of sweeteners include invert sugars and concentrated fruit juice.

Sucrose is made up of two other sugars, glucose and fructose, and comes from processing sugar cane or sugar beets. When unrefined it is brownish in color (turbinado sugar is unrefined sucrose). Refinement removes the color (and the few nutrients still there) to produce the white crystal form of table sugar. Molasses is the least refined form of sucrose and does contain minerals and other nutrients.

Fructose is known as fruit sugar or levulose and is present in fruit. However, the fructose that is added to foods or sold as a sweetener doesn't come from fruit. It's made from sucrose or corn syrup, both already highly refined, by further chemical processing. When added to foods as high-fructose corn syrup it is made from cornstarch. Fructose (as well as sorbitol and mannitol) may have a laxative effect in some people. The fructose content is why apple juice may cause diarrhea in some children (and in some adults). For children who seem to have diarrhea associated with drinking sweetened drinks and fruit juices, it may be a good idea to decrease the amount of fructose-containing drinks and foods with polyols. Fructose can also increase cholesterol levels, especially LDL cholesterol (the "bad" cholesterol). LDL is the type most involved in clogging the arteries, thus increasing the risk of heart disease. And yes, cholesterol is a problem for children. More and more children are found to have high cholesterol levels, while many teenagers already have the beginnings of clogged arteries.

The polyols sorbitol, mannitol, and xylitol are found in fruits, berries, and other plants or are made synthetically. These sweeteners can *reduce* the risk of dental caries. Xylitol, made from birch trees, inhibits bacteria. Xylitol cannot be fermented into acid by mouth bacteria. The bacteria can't use xylitol for energy and thus can't grow. Xylitol also decreases the acidity of the mouth. The greatest benefit is from xylitol-sweetened gum. Chewing it increases saliva flow. Saliva helps clear carbohydrates from the mouth, buffers (decreases) acid levels, and contains minerals that can be deposited in the teeth to strengthen them when acid levels are low. The FDA allows manufacturers to make the health claim that sugar alcohols such as xylitol do not promote tooth decay.

Xylitol can also decrease the occurrence of acute ear infections in children. It inhibits the growth of the bacterium that is one of the major causes of ear infections. In one study, children who used xylitol gum had 45% fewer episodes of ear infection; with xylitol syrup, 32% fewer; and with xylitol lozenges, 22% fewer episodes.

Sweeteners that have calories (and provide energy) are called "nutritive", while those without calories (no energy) are called "nonnutritive."

Stevia is a unique sweetener. It's a natural plant substance that has so far proven safe for everyone, including diabetics, has no calories, and can be used for baking as well as sweetening liquids and foods. It is not a sugar.

When we speak of sugars, however—whether it's honey, fructose, sucrose, corn syrup, maple syrup, or molasses—they are no better (or worse) for you than refined white sugar. All of these sugars play a role in tooth decay, since bacteria in the mouth break down sugar, producing an acid that erodes tooth enamel. But the sugar can just as easily come from the breakdown of starchy foods such as bread and potatoes as it can from candy bars. Sugary foods that stay in your mouth—soft drinks and fruit drinks sipped throughout the day, for example—are worse than sugar added to your morning cereal. Regular brushing and flossing to remove sugar as quickly as possible provides some protection, but there is more to the story.

Sugar Is Not the Whole Story

Way back in A.D. 200 the Greek physician Claudius Galen said, "No cause is efficient without an aptitude of the body." What he meant was that a sickness or disease wouldn't take hold in the body unless the body were weak or susceptible to that disease. The same is true of a tooth. Although many studies show that high-sucrose diets cause dental caries, there is also evidence that enriching these diets with nutrients decreases the number of caries. Ralph R. Steinman, D.D.S., M.S., wrote about the effects of good nutrition on teeth in the *Journal of Applied Nutrition* in 1987.

Dr. Steinman says that the idea that carbohydrates (sugars) are used as food by mouth bacteria which then turn the sugars to acid and dissolve tooth enamel may not be the whole story. It doesn't include what is happening inside the tooth. A good comparison is a plant growing in the ground. If the soil is rich with nutrients, the plant picks them up. Plants grown in healthy soil are better able to resist bugs and other pests. It seems logical that a tooth that picks up good amounts of vitamins and minerals and other nutrients from the bloodstream would also be able to resist disease. This is why we recommend a healthy, nutritious diet for your child.

Tests in animals show that injecting sugar into the bloodstream so that it just gets to the teeth from the blood vessels inside the tooth causes just as much or more caries than having the animal eat the sugar. So sugar can cause caries from the inside or from the outside. Brushing and flossing will get rid of the sugar outside, but doesn't protect teeth from the sugar inside. That is why we recommend limiting sugar in your child's diet. Dr. Steinman's conclusion is that the real story may be that caries are caused by acids produced by the mouth bacteria acting on teeth that are poorly nourished and therefore not able to resist disease.

How Much Sugar Is Too Much?

There is just too much sugar in the average American diet. Americans eat more candy than eggs, drink more sugared soft drinks than milk, and down as much sugar as the combined intake of eggs, all fruits, potatoes, all other vegetables, and whole-grain cereals. The average American eats about 150 *pounds* of sugar a year. Our grandparents' average sugar intake was about 7 pounds per person. Even if you think that you eat only half or a quarter of that amount, that still adds up to 40 to 75 pounds a year. How do we get to such high figures? Look at the sugar content of some often used foods:

SUGAR CONTENT OF COMMON FOODS

Skittles candy (2 oz)	45 grams	11 ¼ tsp
Frosted wheat biscuits (5)	10 grams	2 ½ tsp
Oreos (3)	13 grams	3 ¼ tsp
Cranberry juice cocktail (1 cup)	25 grams	6 ¼ tsp
Chocolate chip ice cream (1 cup)	48 grams	12 tsp
McDonald's vanilla shake	71 grams	17 ¾ tsp
Double fudge brownie (3 oz)	47 grams	11 ¾ tsp

1,000 grams = about 2.2 pounds
1 tsp sugar = 4 grams

Each 5-gram serving of sugar (about a rounded teaspoon) raises a child's risk of caries development by 1%.

Beware of statistics. The National Institute of Dental Research released information that refined sugar consumption decreased by 33% during the 1980s. This sounds like good news for dental health. However, "refined" sugar had been defined by the FDA as sucrose (table sugar from cane or beet), not counting other sugars with calories (also refined) such as high-fructose corn syrup, glucose, dextrose, honey, and other edible syrups. Also omitted were sorbitol and mannitol. According to noted nutritionist Beatrice Trum Hunter, "This limited definition of 'refined sugar' is unscientific, because all caloric sugars are detrimental to teeth."

In case you think it's just Americans that suffer from sugar excess, here is a story that shows that sugar ruins teeth worldwide. "Into the Heart of Africa" by William Carl, D.D.S., was published in the *New York State Dental Journal*. It is an account of Dr. Carl's journey to a tiny village, Houro-Daoudan. It is a 2-hour walk from Djohong, a larger village in Cameroon that is not even on the map. In the smaller village, Dr. Carl, as part of the Earthwatch Community Health Project, examined the teeth of the children. He was pleasantly surprised to see that there was almost no dental decay, but there was a fair amount of gingivitis caused by plaque. Even the adults had very little decay. He showed them how to use fresh sticks from trees and bushes to clean their teeth, similar to the Meswak (Peelu) sticks described in chapter 5. There was no point in giving them toothbrushes since they would be shared by different family members and wear out, with no replacements available. Then Dr. Carl went to the larger town, Djohong, expecting to see the same lack of decay there. He was shocked when he saw the terrible decay in both children and adults. The reason was that these people liked things sweet: coffee, tea, everything is sweetened with sugar. Together with not brushing and the lack of a dentist, their teeth were doomed. They did not even use Meswak.

Liquid Candy

Many people don't count a soft drink as "junk food" simply because it's a drink. It's true it doesn't contain fat, but a Coke or Pepsi or other cola drink is not any better that a whole bag of candy. It's primarily made up of water, colors, and sugars. A can of Coke has 39 grams of sugar (9 ¾ tsp) and a can of Pepsi has 41 grams of sugar (10 ¼ tsp). That's a lot of sugar!

Robert L. Frazer, Jr., D.D.S., writing in the Austin Dental Society newsletter, tells us that dentists are seeing a steady increase of patients with enamel problems ranging from cracking to total tooth erosion. One explanation is excessive consumption of diet soda. Soda consumption in this country is growing. Americans drank an average of 486 cans per person in 1985, up from 289 cans in 1975. This figure has increased by 43% since 1985 to over 690 cans—almost 3 cans a day. And diet sodas accounted for more than 20% of sales. The harmful effects on tooth enamel come from the phosphoric and citric acids that are added to soda as flavor enhancers. In diet sodas, taking out the sugar makes them even more acidic and more harmful to tooth enamel. Experts stress that teeth may be dissolving all over at once in soda drinkers and that changes may not be easily visible to either the dentist or the patient until extensive damage is done.

Hidden Sugar

You may believe that your child eats very little sugar, because when you think of sugar, you think only of the visible kind. What you sprinkle on or stir into foods and even candy is really only a small part of total sugar intake. The greatest amount is in the form of "hidden" sugar. Even if we know the foods that contain sugar, we underestimate just how much they contain. For example: Sugar becomes part of our diet in different ways. It is added during food processing in sweet baked goods, candy bars, snack foods, soda pop, fruit drinks, and cereals and is hidden in many foods such as sweetened fruit juices and granola cereals. It is added during food preparation and at the table in the form of white or brown sugar, maple or corn syrup, molasses, honey, and jam.

About 75% of the sugar we eat is in packaged and prepared foods and beverages. Few supermarket items are free of sugar. We don't buy ketchup because we want sugar. The food industry, however, has discovered that they can sell more ketchup if they spike it with sugar. Other foods that contain sugar are canned meats, soups, and even potato chips. Peanut butter and hot dogs may contain sugar, although you can get them without it. Read the labels. Foods are listed in order of amount in the food: the first ingredient is the highest amount. If sugar (or one of its forms) is listed first, second, or third, you know that there is a lot of sugar or carbohydrate in the food. Such foods should be avoided.

The Center for Science in the Public Interest has the following tips for choosing a good breakfast cereal:

- Ingredients are listed on the label in descending order by amount (the first ingredient is present in the highest amount). If sugar is listed first, reject the cereal.

- Look at the grams of sugar per serving: 6 grams is the maximum recommended by the American Dietetic Association.
- Don't be tricked into buying a sugary cereal with lots of vitamins. The vitamins don't make up for high sugar or additives.
- Look for the words *whole-grain* before ingredients like wheat, rice, corn, or barley.

Sugar also shows up in places not immediately obvious such as in children's medications. Take a look at cough syrups, chewable acetaminophen and prescription medicines. In a study of 769 community pharmacies containing over-the-counter children's medicines (used for treating 12 specific children's ailments), only 2 of the 14 most commonly used medications were sugar-free. Only 1 of the 7 best-selling medications was sugar-free. Seventy-seven percent of the pharmacists believed that sugar in medication could possibly be a factor in dental caries in healthy children. Sugar-sweetened medicines are definitely a problem if given as the last thing at night. It would be equivalent to the "juice bottle" syndrome (tooth decay from putting babies to sleep with bottles).

In a *New York Times* article, we see that drug companies are selling over-the-counter cold and sore throat remedies for children that taste like candy or bubble gum or could be mistaken for ordinary lollipops. Chewy children's acetaminophen now comes in bubble gum, fruit, and grape flavors. Another company is selling lollipops for sore throats while still another has bubble gum for colds. There is even a product for sucking during an asthma attack. The first and most obvious problem is that this is dangerous for children—it's teaching them that medicine tastes good. Says Dr. Sara O'Heron, a maternal-child health specialist at Emory University in Atlanta, "The problem is, on one hand we are trying to make kids distinguish between medicine and candy or food, and now we're blurring that distinction. I think it's a good marketing ploy but it's scary." Some of the products contain potent ingredients that can be harmful to children who mistake them for candy and take too much. One mother said that her 3-year-old who always hated medicine liked the candylike medicine so much that he faked a coughing fit just to get some more.

The second problem is, of course, what the sugar in these "medicines" is doing to children's teeth. This "spoonful of sugar makes the medicine go down" may be fine for Mary Poppins, but it's not so fine for children's teeth. This is not worrying the manufacturers, who are tapping into a $17 billion over-the-counter market where the children's products are growing at a fast rate. The worst offenders are the lollipops and cough drops, because they stay in the mouth the longest.

Even children's vitamin and mineral products may contain sugar. In one study 61% of the products contained sucrose. Parents should look for products made by reputable, health-conscious companies with labels that say that no sugar, artificial colorings, or other additives are in the supplement.

What About Natural Sweets?

Sweet foods can be part of a healthful diet. Moderation is the key. If the sweet foods that have few nutrients don't crowd out the more nutrient-rich foods, they can make eating more interesting. If proper care of your child's teeth goes along with having some natural sweets in the diet, there will be no mouth health problems.

The term *natural* needs some explanation. What food manufacturers mean is that whatever they are calling "natural" was already in the food—and they didn't add it. In the case of sugar, they may say that a box of cereal has "no sugar added." But if you look at the Nutrition Facts label it shows that there are several grams of sugar in the food. What gives? The explanation is that the Nutrition Facts label will list both "naturally occurring" and "added" sugars. Although the words on the box state that no sugar has been added, the cereal contains sources of natural sugar. Many foods, such as fruit, contain natural sugar. Other foods with natural sugar are not as obvious; they include vegetables, milk, grains (as in cereal), and legumes (beans).

If you need to give your child natural sweets, it should be fresh fruit and sweet vegetables such as carrots and sweet potatoes.

These natural sweets are loaded with vitamins, minerals, and other nutrients. They also contain fiber—very helpful in keeping the pancreas from being overburdened with bursts of sugar. Fiber slows the absorption of sugar from the stomach into the blood. The pancreas can then handle the sugar and doesn't have to secrete so much insulin. Fats and protein also slow sugar absorption. An oatmeal cookie, for example, would have oat fiber to slow down the sugar and fat (hopefully the good fats; see chapter 8) to help slow the sugar.

Although all sugars can be used by bacteria to make the acid that causes caries, when it comes to starch the story is not as simple. Whether it will cause caries depends on the type of starch. Cooked or milled starches in foods such as bread, breakfast cereals, and crackers can be used by the bacteria, because they are broken down in the mouth. But the starch in uncooked or lightly cooked vegetables doesn't provide the bacteria with ammunition because very little breakdown of these foods happens in the mouth. Fruit, although healthy in terms of the nutrients it contains, is also broken down in the mouth. So it is recommended that fruits be given in moderation. Rather than take healthy foods such as cereals and fruits out of your child's diet, it is better to practice good dental hygiene.

What About No- or Low-Calorie Sweeteners?

The quick answer is that it's not a good idea to give children no- or low-calorie artificial sweeteners. For one thing, children need the energy that comes from carbohydrates as long as it is not in excess. Also, children's livers and kidneys are immature in their ability to detoxify chemicals compared with adult body systems. Adding nonnatural sweeteners are just adding a chemical burden to your child's detoxifying systems.

The longer answer is that you need some facts to make your own decision as to whether no-calorie or low-calorie sweeteners are better than sugar or worse for your child's teeth and health. The sugar substitutes approved for use in the United States include aspartame, saccharin, acesulfame-K, and sucralose. Artificial sweetener intake went from 5 pounds per person each year in 1970 to 25 pounds in 1991. Saccharin is a noncaloric, indigestible petroleum (yes, the same source that oil and gasoline comes from) product that is 300 times sweeter than sugar. In the late 1970s, a study linked saccharin to cancer in laboratory rats, and the product was nearly removed from the market. But the case against the sweetener was dropped when the researchers said that the rats had consumed saccharin in the equivalent of 800 cans of diet soda a day. There is, however, almost no information about the effects of saccharin in children, so using it is not recommended. Because saccharin can cross the placenta and reach the unborn baby, other sweeteners should be used during pregnancy.

Aspartame is a synthetic combination of two amino acids, aspartic acid and phenylalanine, along with methanol (an alcohol). The amino acids are found naturally in milk, meat, and dried beans, but they are not found together in nature as they are in aspartame. Methanol, although found in small amounts in foods, can become a problem in larger amounts. Methanol is a toxin; another name for it is wood alcohol. Two teaspoons of it is lethal to humans. In the body it breaks down to formic acid (ant sting poison) and formaldehyde, another poison (used to preserve dead bodies). If a child drinks two thirds of a 2-liter bottle of diet soda (which may be possible in hot weather or during exercise), 70 mg of methanol is taken into the child's body. This is about 10 times the Environmental Protection Agency's recommended daily limit of consumption for methanol. Aspartame also increases thirst, making it likely that even more will be taken in. Although the FDA ruled that most people (adults) could safely consume the equivalent of 97 packets of aspartame daily, some consumers have complained of headaches and other side effects. Some people believe that aspartame triggers their migraine headache attacks.

Aspartame was approved in 1981 and by 1984, Woodrow C. Monte, Ph.D., R.D., director of the Food Science and Nutrition Laboratory at Arizona State University, had received over 1,000 written complaints of health problems from people using aspartame. Aspartame was originally approved for use in powdered drinks and as a tabletop sweetener. Aspartame contains 4 calories per gram, just like sugar. But aspartame is 200 times sweeter than sugar, so much less is needed. In 1996, aspartame was approved for use in all foods and beverages, including products such as syrups, salad dressings, and snack foods. All foods containing aspartame must carry a label warning that people with phenylketonuria (PKU), an inherited inability to metabolize one of the amino acids (phenylalanine) in aspartame, should not eat the product. Infants are routinely tested at birth for the presence of PKU since eating foods with phenylalanine can result in brain damage and retardation in these children.

Acesulfame-K is chemically similar to saccharin and 200 times sweeter than sugar. It's found in dry beverage mixes, instant coffee and tea blends, puddings, gelatin mixes, and chewing gum. The sweetener's safety was called into question when laboratory rats developed tumors during testing, but the FDA maintains that the tumors were unrelated to the product.

Sucralose is the only no-calorie sweetener made from sugar. It is about 600 times sweeter than sugar and is used in baked goods, desserts, dairy products, canned fruits, syrups, and condiments. Although scientific studies have shown that it does not cause cancer, remember that scientific studies are rarely done on children. Children's immune systems and detoxification mechanisms are much less effective than those of adults. Sucralose also contains chlorine, which is what makes it pass through the body and not add calories. While chlorine is found in the water we drink and naturally in some foods, the question again is, "Do we need an extra burden of chemicals in our children's bodies?"

Fruit sodas, especially lemon and lime, are usually kept clear and transparent with sugar. In diet sodas, the sugar is replaced by stannous chloride (a form of metal tin) as a clarifier. It's possible for bacteria in the intestine to convert the tin to chemicals that can affect the brain. Manufacturers could use vitamin C, instead, to keep the soda clear; however, it costs slightly more than the tin chemical, so they don't use the safer method of keeping diet drinks clear.

Just remember that none of these artificial sweeteners have had studies done with children to see the effects on their bodies. Children who eat these sweeteners are the guinea pigs right now.

Separating Your Child from Sugar

Why do we have a "sweet tooth"? If you ask a scientist the answer would be that liking sweets has to do with survival. If you give infants a choice of tastes such as sweet, salty, bitter, or sour, the sweet taste is the infants' choice. This may be a genetic design that makes sure that an infant will accept life-sustaining milk from the breast or bottle with its slightly sweet taste that comes from milk sugar (lactose). Many of us, however, go beyond that inherited taste for sweets, because that's what we are used to. In the 1940s, baby food contained sugar. Parents gave babies sugar water when they cried to calm them. Early childhood "rewards" were cookies and candy. Many of these habits were passed on to the next generation. We believe that the baby wants sweet foods, because that is what we like and are used to. Although we know more about sugar and tooth decay today, we are still bombarded with sugar advertisements by the media. This adds to our problem of trying to get sugar out of our diets and that of our children.

It's difficult enough to get your child to brush and floss (or to let you do it). How are you going to get a child who is surrounded by sweets and used to sweets, to cut them out?

> Most people believe that foods containing cholesterol and saturated fats can cause high cholesterol levels and lead to heart disease. Another type of blood fat, the triglycerides, is just as dangerous when elevated as is cholesterol. Triglycerides can be elevated as a result of eating high amounts of fructose and sucrose (about two to three times normal amounts).

If you know that your child is eating sweets, where do you start to reduce the amount of sugar in his or her diet? Start by looking at your child's "sugar habits" and start to change them, one habit at a time. The first group to start with is the foods high in sugar and low in healthy nutrients. These include:

- Soda pop or sweet drinks
- Chocolate bars
- Sweet baked goods such as cookies, pies, cakes, doughnuts, pastries, granola bars, and other sweet desserts
- Sugar that is added to foods such as cereal

Once you eliminate these "foods" or reduce the amount substantially, the next group to work on is the nutritious foods that have added sugar. These should be decreased in your child's diet:

- Sweetened fruit juices
- Sweetened cereals
- Sugar added to fruit
- Syrup added to food
- Jam or jelly used on bread

The idea is to slowly cut back on sugar and gradually allow your child to enjoy foods that are not as sweet. A good rule is to choose sweets that have less than 5 grams of sugar per serving. Replace high-sugar foods with something more nutritious—for example:

- Instead of pop, try water (something that most children get very little of), unsweetened fruit juices (which can be diluted with water), plain soda water, or plain water with a splash of orange or grape juice added.
- Some sugar or syrup to top unsweetened cereals, pancakes, and waffles is okay, but try to cut down gradually. Use fresh or unsweetened frozen fruit as a topping. Unsweetened applesauce, crushed pineapple, strawberries, or blueberries are delicious.
- Add your own fresh, unsweetened canned or frozen fruit to plain yogurt rather than using the highly sweetened fruit-flavored varieties.
- Serve fresh fruit or unsweetened fruit sauce (such as applesauce) for dessert and snacks instead of rich pastries, cakes, and cookies. The whole fruit contains fiber and bioflavonoids (nutrients that work with vitamin C) and much less sugar per serving than fruit juice.
- Choose unsweetened fruit juices or canned fruits packed in water, their own juices, or light syrups. Labels tell you if a juice is sweetened.
- When baking, you can reduce the sugar in a recipe up to one third without ruining the finished product. Extra vanilla or

spices in a recipe enhance sweetness. Serve cakes without icing.

- At snack times, choose whole-grain muffins (bran, oatmeal, whole-wheat), cheese with whole-grain crackers, or fruit bread.
- Make your own muffins without sugar or hydrogenated oils.
- Freeze fruits without adding sugar. Bananas, strawberries, and other fruits can be used to make milkshakes or fruit smoothies.
- Use stevia to sweeten your foods, instead of sugar.

In March of 1999, the Department of Agriculture released the first guidelines on how to feed young children a nutritious diet. The guidelines are in the form of a pyramid (see chapter 8) with grains at the base and a soda can at the top. Soda companies were outraged because soda was singled out as a high-sugar food that shouldn't be used very often. The undersecretary of agriculture for Food, Nutrition and Consumers Services, Shirley Watkins, said that the most a young child should drink is half a 12-ounce can of soda a day. According to Agriculture Department statistics, 37% of children 2 to 6 years of age in the United States drink an average of 10 ounces of soda.

Behavior is closely linked with eating habits. It's easy to figure out what happens to a child's food preferences if he or she is rewarded with sweets. How many times have you heard: "What a good boy, here's a lollipop." Or, when a child is sick: "Here, have a cup of hot chocolate to make you feel better." Even the terms of endearment and praise that we use are full of sugar: "honey," "sweetie pie," "sugar plum," "what a sweet child," "you're sweet as sugar candy," "come give me some sugar"—you can see that it's not an easy job to lower the sugar levels in your child's life!

Timing Is Important

Sugar definitely plays a role in the development of tooth decay. The number of times a day you eat sugar, rather than the amount you eat, is the key. If you decide to give your child sweets, *when* you give them can make a difference in the risk for his or her teeth. The bacteria in the mouth ferment sugars (and other carbohydrates) to produce acid that causes cavities. The acids continue to affect teeth for at least 20 minutes before they are neutralized by saliva and can't do any more harm. So one way to protect the teeth is to limit the amount of time each day that the bacteria get to work on sugars. Remember, the more times your child eats sugary snacks during the day, the more often you feed bacteria. Surveys indicate that most Americans eat five or six times a day. That's five or six opportunities for the bacteria to work. Just when the body gets rid of the acid from one meal or snack, more acid is formed. Besides limiting the number of meals and snacks, researchers recommend drinking water between meals (not soda pop), and saving sweet or acidic beverages for drinking with foods that can buffer (counteract) the acids produced. Protein from dairy products, meat, and beans decreases the total amount of acid produced from a meal. Fat and water both increase the clearance of food from the mouth and so limit exposure to carbohydrates. So if you must give your child dessert, give it after a main meal instead of several times a day between meals. Sweets eaten alone between meals have a more damaging effect than when they are eaten with a meal, followed by water or, even better, by a protein like milk to counteract acid production. And try to brush after each meal or snack. But remember that clean teeth are not the whole story, as Dr. Steinman told us (see above).

The form of food is also important. Solid foods remain on the teeth longer than liquids. Sticky foods are especially difficult to clean from the teeth. Sticky foods that contain sugar, if eaten between meals, are especially bad news for your child's teeth. Between meals, sticky raisins and other dried fruits can do as much damage as taffy candy. If you do choose something sweet and sticky for your child's snack, be sure to brush and floss afterwards.

Here's a snack list from the National Institute of Dental and Craniofacial Research (a division of the National Institutes of Health):

Fresh Fruits and Raw Vegetables	Grains	Milk and Dairy Products	Meats, Nuts, and Seeds
Berries	Whole-wheat	Low or nonfat	Chicken
Oranges	or multi-	milk	Turkey
Grapefruit	grain bread	Low or nonfat	Sliced meats
Melons	or bagels	yogurt	Pumpkin seeds
Pineapple	Unsweetened	Low or nonfat	Sunflower
Pears	cereals	cheeses	seeds
Tangerines	Unbuttered	Low or nonfat	Other nuts
Broccoli	popcorn	cottage	
Celery	Tortilla chips	cheese	
Carrots	(baked, not		
Cucumbers	fried)		
Tomatoes	Pretzels		
Unsweetened	(whole-		
fruit and	wheat and		
vegetable	low-salt)		
juices	Pasta		
Canned fruits	Plain crackers		
in natural	without hy-		
juices	drogenated		
	fats		

So the task may be difficult to eliminate or reduce sugar from your child's diet. But the rewards are great: a healthy mouth and teeth and a strong immune system. These are gifts that will stay with your child for a lifetime.

CHAPTER · 8

Your Child's Diet for Dental Health

Years ago, we attended lectures given by a periodontist, Dr. Anatol Chari, who made nutrition an important part of his practice. Dr. Chari had a very dry sense of humor. He loved to poke fun at dentists who focused on brushing and flossing, using fluoride, and so on. Dr. Chari showed slides of aboriginal peoples with beautiful teeth and pointed out that they had no toothbrushes, no floss, no fluoride, no toothpaste—and no dentists!

What made the difference between the aborigines' teeth and ours? This third-world society ate a diet of natural foods, free of chemicals that interfered with healthy growth and development.

Teeth are living things. They need internal nutrition as well as calcium to keep the outside of the tooth healthy. The outside of a tooth is the enamel. Under this is a layer of the dentin, which is the main support of the tooth. In the center of the tooth is the pulp, the area where the nerve and blood vessels enter the tooth from below. The pulp-dentin complex requires nutrients from the blood stream. Therefore, the blood vessels in the body must be healthy to carry the nutrients to each tooth.

In order for the nutrients to get into the bloodstream in the first place, all food must be digested properly and absorbed into the bloodstream. As we shall see, this process doesn't always go smoothly.

Despite all we know about how to eat properly, children are still eating poorly—and studies show that their diets have been getting worse. Fewer vitamins and minerals are being taken in, suggesting that children are eating higher-calorie, lower-nutrient foods. The vast majority of U.S. children do not meet federal standards for a healthy, balanced daily diet. Only 1% of children meet the RDA; just over 36% eat the recommended three to five servings of vegetables each day; only 26% regularly eat two to four servings of fruit. And 15% of children's daily calorie intake comes from added (non-naturally sourced) sugars.

What Should Children Eat?

In general, children should eat the foods in the USDA Food Guide Pyramid—but with our recommended changes:

1. Five to seven servings* of bread, cereal, rice, pasta. *Note: Although the USDA recommends six to eleven servings, we feel it would be difficult for a child to eat so much and still get in the more important vegetable servings. The USDA's special food pyramid for children (aged 2 to 6) suggests six servings of grains.* (Be sure bread and cereal are whole-grain. Use brown rice which contains more vitamins and minerals, and choose whole-wheat pasta over white flour.)
2. Three to five servings* of vegetables. *For children, the USDA recommends three servings.*
3. Three to four servings* of fruits. *For children, the USDA recommends two servings. We consider this low.*
4. Three servings* of milk, yogurt, or cheese. *For children, the USDA recommends two servings. Because children need calcium for growth, we prefer three servings.*
5. Three to four servings* of meat, poultry, fish, dry beans, eggs, or nuts. *We recommend two to four servings because protein is important for growth and development.*
6. Use sparingly: fats, oils (see the following page), sweets, and bread, pasta, and cereals that are not whole-grain.

*Remember, serving sizes are smaller for children (from 2 to 4 years old) than for adults. For example, ¾ cup of milk is a serving, a quarter of a banana or apple is a serving, ¼ cup cooked green leafy vegetable, or ½ cup raw vegetable is a serving.

In a study of over 3,100 children and adolescents between 2 and 18 years of age in the United States, nearly one quarter of all the vegetables eaten were French fries. Dark green and/or deep yellow vegetable and fruit consumption was very low compared to government recommendations. Only one in five children ate five or more servings of fruits and vegetables per day.

Infants have their own unique nutritional and developmental needs. Therefore, adult dietary guidelines for fat, protein, fiber, sugars, and other nutrients should not be applied to infants and young children.

Good Fats, Bad Fats

The Food Guide Pyramid doesn't make any distinction between good and bad fats and oils. This is unfortunate, because some fats are essential for the healthy growth and development of your child. Although experts disagree about a lot of things, they all agree that *under no circumstances* should fat be reduced for children under the age of 2. Restricting or limiting fat or calories for infants under 24 months severely inhibit their normal growth.

For children age 2 and older, a diet that contains between 20% and 30% of calories from fat is recommended. If you are using a lower-fat diet than this, check that the child's growth is normal and that the child is eating enough food to meet nutrient needs. The fats to limit in children *over* age 2 are the *saturated* fats, which come primarily from animal sources (beef fat, high-fat dairy products). Saturated fats should be no more than 5% to 10% of a child's daily calories, as amounts over 10% can raise cholesterol levels and contribute to heart disease. Scientists are finding fatty deposits in the coronary arteries of children as young as 3 years when they eat high-fat diets and have elevated levels of cholesterol.

Polyunsaturated fats are a better choice. These fats are found in vegetables, fish, corn, cottonseed, sesame, soybean, and safflower oils. In fact, the fats found in fish can actually lower cholesterol. Fish especially high in "good" fats are salmon, mackerel, herring, anchovies, trout, catfish, and sardines. Polyunsaturated fats should make up 8% to 10% of your child's diet.

Monounsaturated fats are the healthiest fats. They are found in olive oil, peanuts, avocados, some nuts, and canola oil. These fats help lower cholesterol. These should make up 10% of your child's daily calories.

Beware of "partially hydrogenated" fats, or "trans-fatty acids," which are added to many foods, including peanut butter and margarine. These harmful, artificially produced fats actually increase cholesterol levels and interfere with the body's use of the good fats.

All Complex Carbohydrates Are Not Created Equal

Parents are told to check the Food Guide Pyramid to discover which foods to accent in their children's diet. Unfortunately, when it comes to carbohydrates, there tends to be a bit of confusion. That's because the Food Guide Pyramid says grain products are good for us. Unfortunately, it does not distinguish between white bread, white rice, and pasta (with few nutrients and almost no fiber) and more nutritious carbohydrates such as 100% whole-grain breads and cereals, brown rice, and whole-grain pasta.

We need the whole grain carbohydrates to provide B vitamins, minerals, and fiber. If these nutrients are refined out of the carbohydrates, they are no better than starch and sugar.

A prime example is commercial breakfast cereals. Manufacturers take out the bran (fiber) and the wheat germ (packed with vitamins, minerals, and protein) and add a few nutrients back, calling the cereal "enriched." If you take out 25 nutrients and put back 4 or 5, is this really "enriched," or is it really "depleted" cereal?

In addition, sugar is routinely added to bread. B vitamins are needed to process the sugar. The B vitamins that are left rush to process the sugar and are not available to be used elsewhere in the body. In addition, because the B vitamins that were originally in bread were removed, there are not enough to handle both the body's needs and sugar metabolism. The body must take the B vitamins from elsewhere such as the brain and liver. As a result, your baby's body will have to "rob Peter to pay Paul."

Whole grains in their natural state are good sources of important nutrients. They are high in manganese (important in processing sugar), vitamin E (which protects our cells from toxicity), and magnesium (needed to produce energy). However, after the bran and germ are removed, white flour contains only a fraction of its original nutrients.

If the white flour is bleached with toxic chemicals (such as chlorine or bromine), this further reduces the nutrient content, besides leaving some questionable chemical products behind. These are just more chemicals that the liver has to detoxify.

In fact, when lab animals were fed white flour after it was bleached, they suffered from stunted growth.

Additives are another problem. These include preservatives, artificial colors and flavors and processing chemicals. In one experiment combining food additives and a low-fiber diet, animals were given just one additive. The result: no visible effect on their health. When two additives were fed, the aminals looked sickly and showed signs of illness. When three additives were given, all of the animals went downhill rapidly and were dead in 2 weeks! However, when the animals were fed the regular daily requirement of fiber, the researcher could largely counteract the fatal result, and the animals remained healthy.

The normal adult requirement for fiber is at least 20 to 30 grams a day—a little less than an ounce. A high-fiber diet contains 25 grams of fiber for every 2,000 calories eaten. American diets typically include only about half the required fiber.

The additives in our foods have supposedly been proven safe by testing them one at a time on animals fed a balanced diet, with adequate fiber. However, most processed foods, such as commercial bread and cereal, contain more than one additive—and government surveys show that most people don't eat enough fiber. You can easily see that such a diet will get us in trouble.

When choosing your family's food, don't be misled by the words *natural, wheat,* or *grain* in the name of the product or in the ingredient list. Many shoppers assume that *wheat* means "whole wheat" and *grain* means "whole grain," especially when there are pictures of grains growing in the field. If you see the words *wheat flour* this actually means white flour (it came from wheat). Another tip-off is when you see that thiamine, niacin, riboflavin, and iron have been added—this is the "enrichment" done to white flour. Color can be misleading: dark "pumpernickel" breads are usually white flour, perhaps with some added whole-grain flour with caramel color added to give the dark appearance. Beware of breads and other baked goods that are made from whole-wheat or whole-grain flour but then are ruined by adding partially hydrogenated oils and artificial preservatives. Some breads are labeled whole wheat, when the whole wheat is only one ingredient, with the rest of the flour being white flour.

If you want to substitute for meat dishes, choose beans. These are high-protein complex carbohydrates that can substitute for animal protein when combined with grains or pasta. Lentils, split peas, garbanzo beans, and all other beans except for green beans are good protein sources when combined with grains. They also have a relatively high amount of fiber. Several vegetables that are high in complex carbohydrates are white potatoes, sweet potatoes, yams, and parsnips. Unlike legumes, however, they are not high in protein or fiber.

In short, eating more complex carbohydrates is valuable only if they are 100% whole-grain foods, legumes, and other high-complex-carbohydrate vegetables. Avoid white-flour products, white rice, and commercial cereals. They not only crowd out more nutritious foods from your child's diet, but also can contribute to blood sugar problems and are more likely to cause tooth decay.

Foods for Healthy Digestion

In order for the nutrients in food (such as protein, carbohydrates, fats, vitamins, and minerals) to eventually get to the teeth or bones or any part of the body, food must be digested and get into the bloodstream. The way that digested nutrients enter the bloodstream is through the *mucosa,* the skin that lines the mouth, throat, esophagus (tube to the stomach), stomach, and intestines. Different nutrients are absorbed at different places along the digestive tract. For example, starches are digested first by enzymes in the saliva.

Proteins are digested in the stomach. For these processes to work properly, a balance is needed in the digestive tract between good bacteria and bad bacteria.

Many different types of bacteria inhabit the digestive tract—some helpful, such as those that make vitamin B_{12}, and some harmful. When the harmful bacteria overgrow, digestive upsets such as diarrhea, constipation, gas, or cramps can follow. The mucosa becomes inflamed, and absorption of nutrients into the bloodstream does not work as well.

The key to preventing these problems and keeping the right balance is to make sure that there are plenty of good bacteria present at all times. These are the lactobacillus bacteria: *Lactobacillus acidophilus, Lactobacillus bifidus,* and other members of the lactobacillus family. These "friendly" bacteria are found in breast milk. Mothers who are breast-feeding should make sure that they have sources of lactobacillus in their diets. For breast-feeding mothers and for children not being breast-fed, these good bacteria can be found in yogurt (with active cultures).

For children with problems digesting milk and milk products, acidophilus can also come from carrots. Carrot acidophilus is available as a supplement (in a powder that can be added to foods). Many children with milk intolerance can eat small amounts of yogurt containing live cultures of lactobacillus without problems. There are also supplements of lactobacillus or non-milk-based friendly bacteria made especially for children.

Another food ingredient that keeps the digestive tract healthy is fiber. This is the type of fiber found in whole grains such as whole wheat and in wheat bran. This type of fiber (called *insoluble* or *indigestible*) acts like a broom, sweeping out the intestine. It also helps stimulate the growth of the good bacteria. Once your child is eating solid foods, he or she should be eating breads, cereals, and crackers that contain whole wheat. (Stay away from pure wheat bran; it's probably too rough to give to a young child.)

Soluble fiber is also important. This type of fiber can stick on to cholesterol and pull it out of the body. Oatmeal and oat bran are good sources of soluble fiber.

Ready for Solids

When will your baby be ready to eat solid foods? Watch for these signals:

- Baby can sit up
- Baby accepts a spoonful of food when offered
- Baby can chew and swallow
- Baby can move food from the front of the mouth to the back with the tongue
- Baby can grasp food

By this time, the intestinal tract has developed enough to protect your baby against infections. There is no longer a complete dependency on the immunity transferred in breast milk. The liver and kidneys are mature enough to handle foods without being stressed.

The Case for—and Against—Commercial Baby Food

Once your baby is ready for solid foods, should you use commercial baby foods? Those little jars of baby food have come a long way. Once, nitrates, monosodium glutamate, and a lot of sugar were regular ingredients in prepared baby food. Today, these have been removed.

But baby foods are still highly processed and can contain refined, low-nutrient ingredients such as white flour and white-flour products. While a mother might think twice about serving canned spaghetti dinner to her family for every meal, the same mother might feed her baby the equivalent in commercial baby food.

Baby foods also contain high levels of fluoride, which can put babies at risk for discolored teeth. Dental researchers at the University of Iowa found that, of the baby foods they tested, cereals, fruits, and vegetables had the lowest levels of fluoride, while ready-to-eat foods with chicken had the highest.

In prepared baby food, starch fillers are also often used. The Food and Drug Administration says that food starches are safe and suitable for use in baby foods but requires that they be listed on the food label. While starches provide an important source of calories for growing infants, foods with natural starches are a better choice

for your baby than processed, added starches. Peas and sweet potatoes contain natural starch. Added flour (corn, wheat, rice) or food
starch may make the baby food "creamy" but will not add to the
nutrient content.

Organic commercial baby food is available in health stores and
in some supermarkets. You can be quite sure these brands will not
contain any additives including pesticides. Babies are much more
susceptible to the toxic effects of pesticides than adults.

There is, however, no reason to feed prepared baby foods to your
child. You can simply prepare regular table food and mash it with
liquid for your baby. Many food processors have small jar attachments to use for making baby food. Blenders or baby food grinders
can also be used. It's best to peel fruits and vegetables unless they are
pesticide-free, and to wash those you can't peel very well. There is a
special liquid soap or spray designed to remove surface contaminants
on produce. Look for it at your health food store or supermarket.

By the time your baby is about 1 year old, he or she should be eating
a good mixed diet that includes:

- 2 or 3 tablespoons of protein (cheese, fish, chicken, meat, tofu,
  yogurt, cooked egg yolk)
- 2 cups of a calcium-supplying food (milk in some form, whether
  cheese, yogurt, breast milk, or formula)
- 2 to 4 servings of grains, pasta, whole-wheat bread or cereal,
  beans, or dried peas
- 2 or 3 tablespoons of vegetables and fruits (leafy greens, yellow
  vegetables, and yellow fruits
- 1 or 2 tablespoons of other fruits and vegetables

Note that serving sizes for babies are a lot smaller than adult servings. For example, ¼ cup of cereal or pasta or half a slice of bread is
a serving. Babies should not eat salty, fried, high-fat, high-sugar,
empty-calorie foods.

If you want to prepare your baby food from scratch, make sure
you're doing it in a clean work area to prevent accidental contamination. Home-prepared baby food should be steamed and then
thoroughly mashed with a fork or a food processor. Parents need to

be cautious of feeding foods that cannot be mashed by the baby's gums and may cause the baby to choke.

Water added to baby food helps make the food the right consistency. Initially a baby's food should be liquid enough to be sucked from a spoon. Texture of the food plays an important role in oral development. As the baby gets older, lumpier foods will encourage chewing. The baby has to learn and master the up-and-down and side-to-side motions of chewing and the manipulation of the tongue to guide foods.

Babies need water for growth and should have a good intake of fluids every day, especially in hot humid weather.

To Snack or Not to Snack?

Because children have high energy needs, they should eat frequently. Three meals and two or three healthful snacks a day will help children meet their daily nutrition requirements. Remember to brush after snacks if possible, especially after sticky, sweet foods. A good rule is to choose a snack that contains enough nutrients to justify its calories. Ideally, snacks should come from the five main food groups: breads, cereals, rice, and pasta; vegetables; fruits; milk, yogurt, cheese; meat, poultry, fish, dry beans, eggs, nuts (for children over 4 years of age). Some snack ideas are:

Fresh fruit
Cereal (unsweetened) with milk and banana
Graham crackers (whole grain)
Yogurt (plain with fresh fruit added)
Raw vegetable sticks
String cheese
Turkey slices
Vegetable soup
Peanut butter and whole-grain crackers with a banana slice instead of jelly

It may be difficult, but it is not impossible to wean children from sugar and refined carbohydrates when they are used to it. The key is to make changes gradually, not all at once. Introduce healthy foods one at a time to replace nutrient-poor foods.

> Poor dental health that comes from a poor diet may slow growth in young children. Researchers believe that serious levels of tooth decay in early childhood may alter eating and sleeping patterns, thereby causing a decrease in weight in older children.

When one of the authors, Jean Barilla, became "enlightened" and switched her children from white bread to whole-grain bread, the initial reaction was, "Yuck." After a while, however, her children said, "Mommy, white bread tastes like nothing. It has no flavor." So tastes are not totally fixed; they can be changed. Children will get to like fresh fruits and juices rather than fruits canned in heavy syrup and sweet punches. Your child will find that when highly sugared foods have been out of the diet for a while, natural sweets will taste sweeter and the overall taste of foods will improve. High sugar decreases the tasting ability of the taste buds on the tongue. Most finicky eaters will eat more when sugar is out of the diet since it also ruins the appetite.

The Importance of Breakfast

The classic Iowa Breakfast Studies (1949–1961) showed that breakfast was important for keeping a stable blood sugar level and preventing sugar cravings. When you and your child go all night without eating and skip breakfast or eat a poor breakfast, blood sugar levels drop. Low blood sugar can cause fatigue, dizziness, poor concentration, and changing vision. In children it may show up as fussiness and temper tantrums. Eating breakfast also resulted in better performance, weight control, and even attitude improvement. Looking at these earlier studies, researchers found that it took from 22 grams to 36 grams of protein to keep the blood sugar level up to a desirable level. This is a lot of protein: a steak-and-eggs meal and more than most people would care to eat. However, the researchers found that the reason so much protein was needed for balance was that the breakfasts contained white bread, sugar, jam, and juice. These can send blood sugar levels on a roller coaster—up and then down. It took a lot of protein to counteract the effect of these sugared foods.

Aside from the effect of all those refined carbohydrates for breakfast on teeth, eating them ruins your child's day. After fasting all night, if all he or she eats is carbohydrates for breakfast, blood sugar levels will drop later in the morning. Having a mid-morning snack won't help. Low blood sugar can make your child nervous and irritable and produce erratic behavior such as mood swings. If your child is in school, he or she won't be able to concentrate and may be a behavior problem or will be sleepy and have trouble paying attention. Then, to feel better, the child will crave and eat sugar and thus get stuck in a vicious circle.

To break the hold of carbohydrates, all you need to do is add protein to breakfast: an egg, some cottage cheese, yogurt, milk— even a tuna sandwich. Make breakfast too good to miss. If your child wants a peanut butter sandwich or grilled cheese, let him or her have it. As long as it's nourishing, it doesn't have to be "breakfast" food. Older children can help make their own "supershakes." These can be combinations of milk, frozen fresh fruits like bananas and strawberries, peanut butter, and protein powder. There are many nutritious protein-based powders for making shakes. They can be made from soy, egg whites, or milk proteins. You can usually get small packages to sample so that your child can find one that he or she likes.

Non–Milk Drinkers: Where's the Calcium?

Some children can't drink milk because of allergies or lactose intolerance. Others just don't like it and refuse to drink milk. How do you get enough calcium into your child for good bone and tooth growth? For those who have allergies, soy-based formula, enriched with calcium, will meet calcium needs. For older children who are weaned, soy milk fortified with calcium can be one of the ways to meet calcium needs. For children who are lactose intolerant, those who have low levels of the enzyme lactase that digests milk sugar (lactose), you may want to try adding acidophilus to the milk. This can be done in the form of plain (preferably organic) yogurt added to the milk (a teaspoon in a bottle of milk). The live acidophilus can break down the lactose, and in many cases the baby or child will be able to drink milk. Acidophilus is also available as a powder, made especially for infants and children, which can be added to milk or other foods. The lactase enzyme can also be added to milk before drinking, or lactose-reduced milk can be used.

There are other good sources of calcium that can be included in your child's diet. Beans, spinach, and broccoli are good sources; oranges contain calcium, and there are calcium-fortified orange juices. Tofu is a good source of calcium and is used to make nondairy cheeses, puddings, and ice cream.

Low-Fat Diets

Some parents wish to reduce their children's risk of developing heart disease later in life and really restrict the fat in the children's diets (10% to 15% of calories from fat). Putting a child less than 2 years of age on a low-fat diet will guarantee that the child will not grow and develop properly. There is just not enough calories for growth. This will be especially true for that child's brain function. Infants and very young children need the essential fatty acids (the building blocks of fats and oils). We cannot make these essential fats but must obtain them from foods. These essential fatty acids (EFAs) are linoleic acid (an omega-6 form) and alpha-linolenic acid (an omega-3 form). The names in parentheses refer to the numbering system for fats.

If your child is overweight and heading for obesity, cutting down on the essential fats is not the answer. Even if your doctor or magazines or newspapers tell you to cut down on your child's fats, don't do it. The key to good health for your child is to cut out the *bad* fats—those that are saturated, such as animal fats and coconut and palm kernel vegetable oils. The other bad fats, even worse for your health than saturated fats, are the partially hydrogenated fats. These are man-made commercially produced fats and oils that have been processed with chemicals. Aluminum, found in high levels in the brains of people with Alzheimer's disease, is often used to process fats and oils. This is done to give the oils shelf life—they don't become rancid as quickly. Partially hydrogenated fats are made into margarine and added to many processed and prepared foods. Just read the labels on the foods that you buy. Partially hydrogenated (or trans fats as they are also called), actually cause the body to make cholesterol and interfere with the body's use of the good fats. They slow metabolism and make it easier to gain excess weight.

Replace the bad fats in your child's diet with the good ones. The good fats are the monounsaturated fats such as olive, canola, peanut, and avocado oils. Fish oils are also important for your child's brain development. Polyunsaturated fats such as corn, soy, sesame, sunflower, and safflower oils can be part of the diet, but in smaller amounts than monounsaturated fats. Fat in the diet is also necessary for us to absorb the fat-soluble vitamins such as E, A, D, and beta-carotene.

> In a survey of 871 children, doctors found that children whose diets provided less than 30% of calories from fat often consumed too little vitamin B_{12}, B_6, E, thiamine, and niacin.

What you want to cut down on for an overweight child are *calories*. You can do this by cutting out junk food and processed fats such as fast food, other fried foods, most packaged foods, and fat-laden cakes and pastries. The way children (and adults) become overweight is that they eat more calories than they burn. But it is not protein or even fatty food that puts on the weight. It is an excess of carbohydrates. When we eat more carbohydrates than we burn up in calories, the excess carbohydrate is turned into fat and stored in the body. So the foods you want to cut down on are breads, cereals, baked goods, rice, pasta, and starchy vegetables like potatoes and peas.

What happens when there are not enough of the essential fatty acids (omega-6 and omega-3) in the diet? Following is a partial list of problems that may arise.

Signs of Essential Fatty Acid Deficiency

Linoleic acid (omega-6) deficiency causes:

Eczemalike skin eruptions
Behavioral disturbances
Excessive water loss through the skin and thirst
Susceptibility to infection
Failure of wound healing
Growth retardation
Heart and circulatory problems

Linolenic acid (omega-3) deficiency causes:

Growth retardation
Weakness
Impairment of vision and learning ability
Motor uncoordination
Tingling sensations in arms and legs
Behavioral changes
Dry skin
Mental deterioration
Low metabolic rate (making it more difficult to lose weight)
Immune system dysfunction

Because the essential fatty acids are so important, talking about them in more detail is a good idea. One of the essential omega-3 fatty acids is docosahexaenoic acid (or DHA). It is very important for brain and retina development as well as for the heart. The brain is about 60% fat. About 40% of this fat is DHA. In the first year of a baby's life, the brain triples in size. It needs a lot of essential fatty acids, especially DHA, for this growth. An omega-6 fatty acid, arachidonic acid (or AA), is also needed for brain development. DHA is made in the mother's body from essential fatty acids that the mother eats and these come from vegetable, seed, and nut oils. The mother can also eat fatty fish (such as mackerel, herring, albacore tuna, salmon, anchovy, and Pacific halibut) and fish oil and get DHA directly (and AA) without having to make it. Infants can't make DHA, so they must get it from breast milk. Since these essential fats are not found in formula, bottle-fed babies should have vitamin drops that contain a source of DHA (such as cod-liver oil).

DHA and AA are not added to formula in this country, although DHA-supplemented formulas can be found in 50 other countries and have been approved by the expert panel of the World Health Organization. In children with dyslexia or attention deficit hyperactivity disorder (ADHD), it has been found that they cannot convert essential fatty acids in the diet to DHA and AA. Giving DHA and AA as supplements has benefited many of these children.

Vegetarian Diets for Infants and Young Children

Vegetarian diets for infants and young children are more common today than ever before. There are many types of vegetarian diets. The most common type of vegetarian is the person that simply avoids red meat. *Lacto-ovo-vegetarians* avoid meat, poultry, and seafood but eat dairy products and eggs. *Lacto-vegetarians* eat dairy foods but no animal protein or eggs. *Vegans,* who avoid all animal foods, are rarer. Some people are vegetarians for religious or cultural reasons; others choose vegetarian eating patterns for their "health benefits." Whatever the case, parents who consume vegetarian diets often feed them to their infants as well.

In addition to limiting or not eating animal foods, some vegetarians may restrict other foods, or eat only natural or organic foods. Some vegetarian parents may also feed their children special health foods or vitamin supplements, because they want their children to have health advantages. Children of vegan vegetarian parents may be nursed longer.

Since many vegetarian parents were raised as omnivores (eating all foods, including meat), they may not know how to feed their children vegetarian diets. A vegetarian diet that keeps an adult in good health may not be healthy for a small child.

The key to good vegetarian nutrition for children is planning meals. There must be enough energy (calories) and protein to ensure growth and development. Planning also ensures that there are enough vitamins and minerals in the diet and the right amount of dietary fiber. Infants and young children cannot eat as much fiber as adults. Children fed vegetarian diets designed for their needs at each age thrive and enjoy excellent health.

Breast milk, the best food for infants, is the vegetarian infant's diet throughout the first year of life. Vegetarian mothers often continue breast-feeding well into the second year.

For mothers who do not breast-feed, commercial infant formulas based on cow or soy milk may be used and usually permit good infant growth. Whole or low-fat milks, soy milks, and soy drinks cannot be given to infants, because they lack many important nutrients and are poorly digested by small infants. Honey and corn syrup should be avoided if homemade formulas are used, since the spores of the bacterium *Clostridium botulinum* (which can cause life-threatening disease) have been reported in some batches.

Vegetarian mothers produce the same amount of milk as that of nonvegetarians, but there may be some important nutrient differences in the milk. The vitamin D content of breast milk depends in part on what the mother eats. If vegan women eat a diet with very low amounts of vitamin D, especially if they live in cold climates, are African American, or use sun block on their skin (so that little of the pro vitamin in the skin is converted into vitamin D), the vitamin D content of their milk will be especially low. Vitamin D in the "pro" form has to be activated by sunlight before it can work to help calcium get absorbed into bones and teeth. Therefore a vitamin D supplement should be given to the baby throughout the nursing period.

Vitamin B_{12} is also lower in the milk of vegetarian women who breast-feed. The amount of B_{12} is usually enough for the first few months of life, but after the first 4 to 6 months a vitamin B_{12} supplement may be needed. The need for vitamin B_{12} can be met from fortified soy or cow milk formula, and from fish, milk products, and eggs later in infancy. Therefore, even if other sources like lean meat and liver are not consumed, lacto-vegetarians can easily meet their children's B_{12} needs.

Vegetarian children tend to have lower birth weights and are slightly smaller. A study showed that nutrients low in vegetarian diets include iron, vitamin B_{12}, vitamin D, taurine, and omega-3 fatty acids.

All infants, including vegetarian infants, need to have their growth monitored. Since most vegetarian infants are breast-fed, their growth can be compared to nonvegetarian breast-fed infants. Weight gains are a little lower in breast- as compared to bottle-fed infants, but this is normal. It's very important that the infant gets enough calories if he or she cannot be breast-fed, or becomes ill.

Early weaning of young infants from breast or bottle feeding to vegan diets should be avoided, because vegan diets are often very low in calories (energy) and high in bulk and volume. Breast feeding or use of a commercial infant formula (either cow's-milk- or soy-based) should be continued until 1 year of age. Plain soy and cow's milk should not be given until the second year because these milks are poorly digested and may cause occult (not visible) gastrointestinal bleeding and possible allergies, even after early infancy.

Once the baby is weaned from breast milk or formula and foods are introduced, a lot of consideration needs to be given to adding protein sources in the vegetarian infant's diet. The most important consideration is to ensure that energy needs are met so that dietary protein is not burned for energy. Protein is needed to build muscle and other body tissues. Since milk and egg proteins complement cereal-based proteins well, protein quality is not a concern as long as breast milk or infant formula constitutes a fair amount of the infant's diet, or if the infant is fed a lacto-ovo-vegetarian diet.

Problems can arise if infants are weaned to diets consisting only of plant foods, which are low in calories, and when breast milk or formula is not continued, or are just a small part of the diet so that they are nutritionally meaningless. For a protein food to be "complete" it has to contain all the essential amino acids (building blocks of proteins). There are 22 amino acids that we need to keep the body running. We can make only 13 of them in our bodies. We need the others from our diet. These essential amino acids are histidine, isoleucine, leucine, lysine, methionine, phenylalanine, threonine, tryptophan, and valine. Complete proteins are necessary for growth. If one food doesn't have all the essential amino acids, it can be combined with another food that has the missing amino acids. For example, grains are low in the amino acid lysine, but other plant foods higher in lysine, such as legumes (beans or peas) or animal proteins, when combined with the grains, can make a complete protein. The amino acids found in soy and in quinoa, a seed grown in South America, however, are nutritionally equivalent to animal protein (they are complete proteins). Vegetarian diets very high in legumes, particularly whole or nearly whole beans with tough outer skins, may be hard for a child to digest. For the child to get the protein from beans, they need to be well mashed. The best way to ensure that your child gets complete proteins is to include some animal foods, such as human milk or infant formula, each day. It is not necessary to feed your child proteins from different plant foods together in each meal—giving them over the day at different meals will provide complete protein.

Growth problems are greatest among weanlings 4 to 6 months or older who are fed vegan or near vegan diets. Failure to thrive is of special concern for these infants if weaned too early from the breast. The use of a bulky, low-calorie, high-fiber diet at weaning means that the infant would have to eat more than its stomach capacity to get enough nourishment. The American Academy of Pediatrics recommends that daily fiber intakes not exceed 0.5 gm per kg of body weight.

If the diet is poorly planned, there may be deficiencies of nutrients such as vitamins D, B_{12}, calcium, iron, and zinc. Lack of these nutrients affects infant growth and psychomotor (brain and muscle) development. These deficits can be overcome by giving the infant appropriate vitamin and mineral supplements or nutrient-fortified foods.

After 6 to 8 months of age additional plant and animal foods may be added, such as soft fruits and vegetables, eggs, other protein-rich foods, legumes, and green leafy vegetables. Older infants need to eat meals and snacks about four to six times a day in addition to breast feeding.

Until the teeth come in, some plant foods should be avoided. These include wheat germ, granola-type cereals, and other hard foods unless they are mashed. Also, whole nuts and fruits with seeds or pits should be avoided until after the third birthday to prevent choking risks. Infants continue to need relatively high-fat diets throughout the weaning period, and therefore fat intakes should not be restricted.

By the last part of the first year of life, the baby is ready for combinations of foods that provide extra calories, protein, and other nutrients. Some popular combinations are legume and grain mixtures, milk and milk products with grains and green leafy vegetables, and eggs with grains and green leafy vegetables. Legumes can be cooked and mashed and moistened with milk or formula. Nut butters are also good choices. Emphasize mixtures that provide a balanced pattern of essential amino acids and adequate calories to support growth.

After 1 year of age, when children are eating foods other than breast milk or infant formula for the majority of their nutritional needs, thoughtful meal planning becomes essential for ensuring adequate nutrition.

Whole milk and fortified soy milk or soy drinks are good choices for keeping calcium intakes up in the vegetarian toddler's diet. Other calcium-rich foods, such as calcium-fortified juices, can also be included. However, they are no substitute for milk or fortified soy milk since they do not provide the important nutrients phosphorus, riboflavin, and vitamin D.

Whole-grain, home-prepared, lightly milled cereals that are very high in phytates (natural compounds that bind to zinc) can prevent or decrease zinc absorption from milk or formula. Therefore, more highly refined cereals (in this case non-whole grain), milk, soy, nut butters, and legumes should be emphasized in the vegetarian toddler's diet.

Even in nonvegetarian women, there is not enough vitamin D in breast milk to meet the toddler's needs. Therefore, either 10 micrograms of a vitamin D–fortified formula or a vitamin D supplement should be given to the child. Vegetarian children rarely have problems getting enough foods rich in vitamin A sources since dark-green and deep-yellow or orange vegetables provide plenty of these nutrients and are usually emphasized. After 1 year of age, dark-green vegetables are good sources of vitamin A and vitamin C and also provide some calcium.

Vitamin B_{12} is lower in the milk of vegan or near vegan women than in omnivorous women who breast-feed. Therefore, a vitamin B_{12} supplement is needed for breast-fed vegan toddlers. The need for vitamin B_{12} can also be met from fortified soy or cow's milk formulas, from fish, milk products, and eggs. Contrary to the views of many vegetarians, seaweed, spirulina, and other plant foods do not provide vitamin B_{12} reliably or in a form that humans can use. Vitamin B_{12} supplements are not needed for lacto-ovo-vegetarians.

Folic acid is adequate in breast milk up until about 1 year of age, but after that some other dietary sources must also be found. Dark-green leafy vegetables, wheat germ, yeast and other foods high in folic acid can be added to the toddler's diet. Folic acid deficiency has been reported in a few cases of children fed goat's milk as the exclusive source of milk in early infancy. However, in older infants and young children pasteurized goat's milk is a satisfactory source of calcium and other nutrients.

The need for dietary supplements varies, depending on age and dietary pattern. For vegan vegetarian children, if food sources of iron, calcium, zinc, vitamin B_{12}, and vitamin D rich foods are not included, consider a vitamin/mineral supplement containing at least the Recommended Dietary Allowances. Lacto-ovo-vegetarian children usually do not require supplements as long as food iron sources are adequate.

Vegetarians usually feed their children diets relatively low in sodium, since they avoid many high-salt processed foods and meats. Those who make their own baby foods need to remember that adding salt or using foods that are naturally high in sodium such as soy sauce, sea salt, and miso soup will increase their children's sodium intakes.

Finally, vegetarian children are often slightly lighter than non-vegetarians. As long as growth rate is satisfactory and weight remains in the normal range, this is no cause for concern.

Vegan Diets for Infants and Children

Vegan diets do not include any animal products—no eggs or dairy products. Many members of the Vegetarian Resource Group, a vegan organization, have children that are healthy and that grow normally. They do admit that it takes time and thought to feed vegan children. They also agree that the best early food for a vegan baby is breast milk. There are many benefits for the infant that is breast-fed including those for the immune system. As we mentioned in chapter 3, breast feeding helps the infant's immune system, protects against infection, and reduces the risk of allergies. Like other whole, natural foods, it may contain substances needed by growing infants that are not even known to be essential and are not included in infant formulas.

Some nutrition experts do not recommend vegan diets to children under age 5, who may be at risk for anemia, B_{12} deficiency, rickets, and delayed development on such a diet. Vegan diets may also be unhealthy for pregnant or breast-feeding women, who have a greater need for protein, calcium, iron, and calories. If you choose to breast feed, be especially careful that you are getting enough vitamin B_{12}. The body uses B_{12} to form red blood cells, make genetic material, and maintain the myelin sheaths that protect nerve cells. B_{12} deficiency can cause serious nerve damage, so vegans should take a multivitamin or ensure that their diet contains cereals and other products fortified with the vitamin. If your diet does not contain reliable sources of vitamin B_{12}, your breast-fed infant should receive supplements of 0.4–0.5 micrograms of vitamin B_{12} daily. Folate (folic acid), because it is proven to prevent birth defects, must be part of the diet for any woman (vegan or not) planning to conceive or who is pregnant. All women need 0.4 mg daily. If kale and other leafy vegetables are part of the daily diet, the requirement can be met. To be absolutely sure of getting the right amount, a supplement can be taken. The recommended amount of folic acid for a pregnant woman is 0.8 mg daily.

Vitamin D can be made in the skin that is exposed to sunlight. See that your infant gets at least 30 minutes of sunlight exposure per week if wearing only a diaper or 2 hours per week fully clothed without a hat to maintain normal vitamin D levels. However, you should protect your infant's eyes from direct sunlight. Infants' and young children's eyes are more susceptible to the damaging rays of the sun that lead to cataracts in later life. Dark-skinned infants require greater sunshine exposure. If sunlight exposure is limited, due to factors like a cloudy climate, winter, or being dark-skinned, infants who are solely breast-fed should receive vitamin D supplements of at least 5 micrograms (200 IU) per day. This is the amount needed to build bones and teeth and to maintain blood levels of calcium. Vitamin D deficiency leads to rickets (soft, improperly mineralized bones). Human milk contains only very low levels of vitamin D.

The RDA for calcium for women who are pregnant or breast feeding is 1,000–1,500 mg daily. Some plants, spinach for example, contain oxalic acid and other components that inhibit calcium absorption. The calcium in kale and some other vegetables is not absorbed as well as that found in dairy products. Citrus fruits or juices increase absorption of calcium.

There are two forms of iron. Heme iron, the form found in meat and other animal products, is readily absorbed by the body. Nonheme iron, the form found in plant foods such as dried beans, dried fruits, grains, beets, and fortified flour and cereals, is easily inhibited by substances in foods. It is not absorbed into the bloodstream and anemia may result. Foods high in tannins or caffeine, such as tea and coffee, inhibit iron absorption. Ascorbic acid (vitamin C) actually helps iron to be absorbed more easily. The iron content of breast milk is generally low, no matter how good the mother's diet is. The iron in breast milk is readily absorbed by the infant, however. The iron in breast milk is adequate for the first 4 to 6 months or longer. Recommendations call for use of iron supplements (1 mg/kg/day) beginning at 4–6 months to ensure adequate iron intake.

If you choose not to breast-feed or if you are using formula to supplement breast feeding, there are several soy-based formulas available. These products support normal infant growth and development. Soy-based formulas are used by vegan families as the best option when breast feeding is not possible. At this time all soy formulas contain vitamin D derived from lanolin (sheep's-wool oil). Some soy-based formulas may contain animal-derived fats, so check the ingredient label. Soy formulas can be used exclusively for the first 6 months. Iron supplements may be needed at 4–6 months if the formula is not fortified with iron.

Soy milk, rice milk, and homemade formulas should not be used to replace breast milk or commercial infant formula during the first year. These foods do not contain the right amounts of protein, fat, and carbohydrate, nor do they have enough of many vitamins and minerals for your baby's nutritional health.

It is a good idea (whatever the diet type) to introduce one new food at a time so that any allergies can be later identified. Many people use iron-fortified infant rice cereal as the first food. This is a good choice as it is a good source of iron, and rice cereal is least likely to cause an allergic response. Cereal can be mixed with expressed breast milk or soy formula so the consistency is fairly thin. Formula or breast milk feedings should continue as usual. Start with one cereal feeding daily and work up to two meals daily or ⅓ to ½ cup. Oats, barley, corn, and other grains can be ground in a blender and then cooked until very soft and smooth. These cereals can be introduced one at a time. However, they do not contain much iron, so iron supplements should be continued.

When cereals are well accepted, fruit, fruit juice, and vegetables can be introduced. Fruits and vegetables should be well mashed or pureed. Mashed banana is one food that many infants especially enjoy. Other fruits include mashed avocado, applesauce, and pureed canned peaches or pears. Citrus fruits and juices are common allergens and should not be given until the first birthday. Mild vegetables such as potatoes, carrots, peas, sweet potatoes, and green beans should be cooked well and mashed. There is no need to add spices, sugar, or salt to cereals, fruits, and vegetables. Grain foods such as soft, cooked pasta or rice, soft breads, dry cereals, and crackers can be introduced as the baby becomes better at chewing. By age 7–8 months, good sources of protein can be introduced. These include well-mashed cooked dried beans, mashed tofu, and soy yogurt. Children should progress from mashed or pureed foods to pieces of soft food. Smooth nut and seed butters spread on bread or crackers can be introduced after the first birthday.

Many parents choose to use commercially prepared baby foods. There are products available for vegan infants. Careful label reading is recommended. Since commercial products contain limited selections for the older vegan infant, many parents prepare their own baby foods. Foods should be well washed, cooked thoroughly, and blended or mashed to the right consistency for the child. Home-prepared foods can be kept in the refrigerator for up to 2 days or frozen in small quantities for later use.

It makes sense for vegans to continue breast feeding for a year or longer, if possible, because breast milk is a rich source of nutrients. Vegan infants should be weaned to a fortified soy milk containing calcium, vitamin B_{12}, and vitamin D. Low-fat or nonfat soymilks should not be used before age 2. Rice milks are not recommended as a primary beverage for infants and toddlers as they are quite low in protein and energy (calories).

The best way to ensure that children grow properly is to make sure that they have enough calories and protein. Some vegan children have difficulty getting enough calories and protein because of the sheer bulk of their diets. Children have small stomachs and can become full before they have eaten enough food to sustain growth. Fiber may limit the amount of food they can eat. The fiber content of a vegan child's diet can be reduced by giving the child some refined grain products, fruit juices, and peeled vegetables. The use of fats in forms like avocados, nuts, nut butters, seeds, and seed butters will provide a concentrated source of calories needed by many vegan children. Dried fruits are also a concentrated calorie source and are an attractive food for many children. Teeth should be brushed after eating dried fruits to prevent tooth decay.

Are very-low-fat diets appropriate for vegan children? There is no evidence that a very-low-fat diet is any healthier for a vegan child than a diet that has somewhat more fat (20% to 30% of calories from fat).

Sources of protein for vegan children include legumes, grains, tofu, tempeh, soy milk, nuts, peanut butter, tahini, soy hot dogs, soy yogurt, and veggie burgers. Some of these foods should be used daily. Children should get enough calories so that protein can be used for growth in addition to meeting energy needs.

Although today more and more children are vegans from birth, many older children also become vegan. There are many ways to make a transition from a nonvegan to a vegan diet. Some families gradually eliminate dairy products and eggs, while others make a more abrupt transition. Regardless of which approach you choose, be sure to explain to your child what is going on and why, at your child's level. At first, offer foods that look familiar. Peanut butter sandwiches seem to be universally popular (beware: some kids are allergic to peanut butter), and many children like pasta or tacos. Gradually introduce new foods. Watch your child's weight closely. If weight loss occurs or the child doesn't seem to be growing as rapidly, add more concentrated calories and reduce the fiber in your child's diet.

Junk Food and Soft Drinks

The best way to protect your child's teeth and body from junk food is never to feed these foods. Parents are the most important role models that children have. Their likes and dislikes about food will reflect your preferences. If they hear you say that yogurt is "sour" or broccoli has a "strong" taste, they will adopt the same beliefs. If they see you enjoying fresh fruit or munching on carrot sticks, they will think this is the natural way to eat. The alternative to giving your child good eating habits is something we've all seen: a child in the supermarket screaming for sugar-laden breakfast cereal while the mother tries to quiet him down with cookies or candy.

What do you do around the holidays when "all the other kids" are eating candy and other sweets? According to *Prevention* magazine adviser Dominick DePaola, D.D.S., Ph.D., some sweets are worse than others. The sugar-and-starch combination such as caramels, marshmallows, and gumdrops makes a good meal for cavity-inducing bacteria. He believes that eating sweets for dessert right after a meal will cause less decay. This is because the foods in the meal dilute the acid that forms when sweets are eaten. A small chunk of cheese can decrease the effect of the sugar. Monterey Jack, Muenster, and Cheddar are good choices for children, according to Dr. DePaola. For older children, peanuts and popcorn are good snacks with much less potential for tooth decay.

Little Caffeine Addicts

A study published in the *Journal of the American Academy of Child and Adolescent Psychiatry* (Aug. 1998) examined the effects of caffeine on children. When children who had been getting about 146 mg of caffeine a day for 13 days (equal to three cans of caffeinated soda a day) went "cold turkey," their attention in a performance test dropped because they were restless and irritable. Caffeine is also a diuretic and washes out important minerals such as calcium, magnesium, and zinc. NOTE: There is caffeine in many foods: one cup of coffee-flavored ice cream or frozen yogurt contains up to 85 mg of caffeine; one cup of hot chocolate has 5 mg; a 1.5-oz chocolate bar has 10 mg.

Beware of Sports Drinks

Some parents may give their children sports drinks, thinking they are good. However, when eight sports drinks (including Gatorade and Carbolode) were tested for acidity, all were acidic enough to erode tooth enamel. Fresh fruit juices and carbonated drinks including soda pop also are acidic. To reduce the potential for damage from these acidic beverages, dentists recommend chilling them thoroughly, because the chemical reactions that erode teeth occur more slowly at cooler temperatures. In addition, drinking them through a straw helps keep the teeth's contact with the liquid to a minimum, which may help reduce tooth erosion. A better, low-acid drink is one part fruit juice with four parts water.

Soft Drinks, Soft Bones?

Soft drinks deserve special mention when talking about junk foods that are harmful to your child's health. In one study, a diet high in sugary sodas and low in leafy greens and whole grains was found to have a bad effect on calcium levels in teenaged boys. The USDA found that drinking less than five cans of soda a day over a period of several weeks decreased calcium and phosphorus levels. The effects on these bone minerals were greater if their diets were low in magnesium (found in leafy greens and whole grains). In another study, samples of Coca-Cola (and canned lemon juice) were incubated (mixed together) with human teeth for 15 minutes, 45 minutes, or 12 hours. All teeth examined under a microscope showed an irregular loss of enamel, a loss of gloss, and a change in color. The erosion of enamel got worse the longer the teeth were in contact with the soft drink. This shouldn't come as a surprise to people who have used Coca-Cola as a solvent for cleaning their pennies. In addition to the large amounts of caries-producing sugar in cola beverages (more than 8 teaspoons per 12-ounce can), the phosphoric acid in colas makes these beverages strongly acidic (almost as acidic as lemon juice). Advice was given to rinse out the mouth or brush the teeth after drinking colas (or lemonade).

Does Your Child Need Dietary Supplements?

Dietary deficiency diseases can show up as symptoms (like sores) in the mouth. The tissues inside the mouth act like mirrors that show changes such as vitamin deficiencies, often before there are any other signs. Cells that divide and grow rapidly, such as those that line the cheeks and the inside of the lips, show deficiencies early on because they are using up nutrients very quickly. Almost all of the classic nutritional deficiency diseases, such as scurvy (vitamin C deficiency) and pellagra (vitamin B_3 or niacin deficiency), as well as a host of immune deficiencies, have signs and symptoms in the mouth. The cheek linings may have sores that are slow to heal, there may be fissures or cracks in the lips and tongue, gums may bleed easily, and teeth may become loose in their sockets. A steady supply of vitamins, minerals, and other nutrients are needed for cells to grow and be replaced, for repairs (such as healing) to take place, and for the immune system to fight infections.

It's important for the skin that lines the mouth (mucosa) to be healthy, because it acts as a first line of protection against viruses, bacteria, yeast, and parasite infections. These microbes produce toxic substances, which further injure the tissues and can even destroy the underlying connective tissues that support the teeth. So you can see that it's important to have the best nutrition for your child that produces oral health.

Does your child need supplements of vitamins and minerals for optimal health? The answer will depend on several things. Infants usually get all the nutrients they need from breast milk and most of what they need from infant formula. However, when a child starts eating solid foods, he or she is liable to become finicky or have difficulty eating when teething. So experts say that you don't need to give children vitamins and minerals until they begin eating solid foods. They believe in giving a multivitamin each day because most children don't eat a balanced diet. Although many experts, such as Kathi Kemper, M.D., author of *The Holistic Pediatrician* (Harper-Collins), say that a balanced diet (without supplements) is best, she also says that relatively few children meet the daily RDA for vitamins and minerals.

When choosing a multiple vitamin supplement for your child,

some good advice to remember is that the more natural the ingredients, the better. Some brands contain additives such as starch, yeast, food coloring, and the chemical sweetener aspartame (see chapter 7). It is especially important to read labels and stay away from yellow dyes (see below). No supplement will do your child any good if he or she won't eat it. You may have to try a few brands before you find one that your child likes. Many health food stores have samples of children's vitamins on the counter since they are aware of this problem. Children under 3 may choke on chewable tablets, so it's best to stick to liquids for them. You can mix liquid vitamins with fruit juice. It's very important not to give children adult supplements; the doses are too high, and the pills may be too big to swallow.

Sugar and Harmful Additives Cancel Out the Benefits of Supplements

If you are feeding your child nutritious foods and adding supplements as needed, you don't want to cancel these beneficial effects on his or her health. However, that's just what sugar in excess and harmful food additives do. In order for the body to metabolize or process sugar, it uses B vitamins. The body will take these B vitamins from the food coming in and they will not be available for other important processes in the body. Breaking down and getting rid of the sugar will use them up. If the diet is low in B vitamins (which are found in whole grains and brown rice, meat, and dairy products) then the body will "borrow" B vitamins from other places in the body. The brain uses B vitamins and a deficiency will cause poor brain function: lack of concentration, nervousness, and so on. Or the body will borrow B vitamins from the liver. The liver uses B vitamins to help detoxify any harmful substances that get into the body. So besides preventing tooth decay, eating less sugar will help the body function at its best.

The same is true of harmful food additives or environmental toxins. The body uses a lot of vitamins and minerals to detoxify these substances. The body enzymes that do the detoxification process need B vitamins, antioxidants (such as vitamins E, C, and beta-carotene) and minerals such as zinc and selenium to do their job. So if you use up the nutrients in the food you eat to get rid of the additives, then the food is really not providing any nutrients. For example, if you eat corn, which contains beta-carotene, and then put margarine on it (containing trans-fatty acids), the beta-carotene is used up to detoxify the trans-fatty acids; there is no beta-carotene left for the body to use in other ways. Another example is a child's multivitamin supplement. If the supplement contains sugar, artificial colors and flavors, and preservatives, then the body will use up all of the vitamins and minerals to detoxify the unwanted ingredients. It will be the same as if you didn't give your child a multivitamin (although you paid for it).

Researchers looking at the content of children's vitamins found that sucrose was present in 61% of the products, FD&C Yellow#6 in 46%, FD&C Red #40 in 29%, and FD&C Blue #2 in 22%. Other chemicals included talc, silicon dioxide, alcohol, propylene glycol, benzoic acid, and polysorbate 80. Some of these chemicals were not listed on the label and were discovered only by contacting the manufacturer directly and asking about unlisted ingredients.

Some additives to beware of:

Nitrates or nitrites.   These substances are found in hot dogs, bacon, and cold cuts. These additives can form cancer-causing substances called nitrosamines. Vitamin C protects against this formation and is used up doing so.

Olestra.   A "fake fat" that tastes like the real thing but has no calories is being added to potato chips, ice cream, and other high-fat foods. In addition to causing diarrhea, cramping, and other side effects in some people (including children) it also sticks to and sweeps carotenoids out of the body. This loss includes beta-carotene and other yellow, orange, or red pigments found in many fruits and vegetables. Carotenoids shield against infections, cancer, and eye problems.

Monosodium glutamate (MSG).   This "flavor enhancer" is added to many foods. It used to be routinely added to Chinese food in restaurants. It is also found in many soups and processed foods.

Many people are sensitive to it and get numbness in the back of the neck, arms, and back, have heart palpitations, or get migraine headaches. It may also trigger asthma attacks in some people.

Research on MSG appeared in the 1950s and 1960s. Researchers found that MSG causes brain and eye damage in newborn rats and mice and in infant monkeys. The Glutamate Association, which represents the MSG industry, claims that MSG can't cross the blood-brain barrier and can't get into the brain. This may not be the case because the barrier is weaker in infants than in adults. Because of public pressure, the baby food industry stopped putting MSG into baby foods. Pregnant or nursing mothers may pass MSG to their babies, so it should be eliminated from their diets. Other research suggests that MSG may work on the area in the brain that controls appetite, causing people not to feel satisfied after eating. Then they overeat and become obese.

Artificial colors. U.S. Certified, FD&C, or USDA approved food colorings are not safe just because they have been approved by government agencies. Remember that this is the same government that knows tobacco is extremely addictive and harmful to your health and still allows it to be sold. Many dyes that were used for years were later found to cause cancer. Artificial colors, besides stressing detoxification systems, cause problems for many children who are allergic to them.

The worst of the artificial dyes is FD&C Yellow Dye #5 (tartrazine). It causes itching, hives, nasal congestion, or headaches in sensitive individuals. A food may not look yellow, so you have to read the label to know for sure. Another name for these yellow dyes is azo dyes. This name refers to the chemical azo group that is part of the dye. Azo groups are very reactive with everything they come in contact with. They cause reactions in the body that destroy cells and use up antioxidant vitamins. Phenolphthalein, a dye related to tartrazine and derived from coal tar, is used to make candy pink. It can produce headaches, breathing difficulties, and other physical problems.

Sulfites. These chemicals are added to foods to keep them looking fresh and to stop spoilage. They were used at salad bars for several years until there were several bad experiences, including deaths, that led the FDA to forbid sulfite spray on fresh fruits and vegetables sold or served raw. Because of their side effects, food labels must list sulfites. Eating sulfites causes mild to severe breathing difficulties in about 5% of people with asthma, or over a million Americans. Symptoms of sulfite reactions are flushing, faintness, weakness, cough, and turning blue. Nonasthmatics can also have symptoms, but they are less severe.

Pesticides

In 1989, the Environmental Protection Agency (EPA) admitted that pesticides found on produce were the third highest threat of environmentally induced cancer, after cigarette smoke and radon. What is even worse is that children are at higher risk than adults are because they eat up to six times more fruits and vegetables than adults. Children also weigh less, so pesticides are present in higher concentrations in their bodies. With immature livers and kidneys, the detoxification ability of children is also less than for adults. The FDA inspects less than 1% of the nation's food supply each year, and it tests for only about half of the 50,000 pesticides currently in use. Even when the FDA rules that a pesticide should be taken off the market, it can remain in use for years while the manufacturer appeals the FDA rulings.

These statistics make a good case for feeding your child organic foods if at all possible. Although organic fruits and vegetables used to be expensive, that is not always the case today. Supermarkets that used to devote one shelf to organic produce now have whole aisles of pesticide-free fruits and vegetables. Because more people are buying organic produce, more farmers are growing chemical-free food; prices are coming down. What can you do if you can't afford to buy organic? There are some alternatives. First, you can buy some things organic—those food items that your child eats all the time and in large amounts. For example, you can buy organic dairy products: milk, butter, cream cheese, and eggs. If your child likes sweet potatoes, buy them organic. Even if you reduce only some of the toxic burden on your child, he or she will be healthier.

Some supermarkets carry what is called "certified residue-free produce." While not necessarily organic, these products are less toxic. They may have been grown with chemicals, but with as few as possible. The chemical residue is certified to be minimal. If organic or residue-free produce is not available, you can make existing foods safer. First, wash all hard-skinned fruits and vegetables thoroughly. Most farm chemicals are oily and will not wash off with a quick rinse under the faucet. Plain soap (made for washing food) and warm water should be used. When possible, peel the fruit or vegetable. Buy fruits and vegetables in season. Especially if locally grown, they will contain fewer chemicals because farmers don't have to add chemicals for shipping.

School Lunches

The idea that children should have a nutritious, hot lunch at noon has fallen short of its original purpose. Due to many factors, including economics, school lunches usually make a questionable contribution to a child's dental and physical health. A glance at a school lunch menu will often reveal an overabundance of cheap, starchy foods and a sugar-laden dessert. The meat and vegetables are usually unappetizingly prepared; a visitor to a school lunchroom will probably see many children eating only the bread, potatoes, and dessert from their lunches.

In one study done about school lunches, it was found that many of today's school menus are built around fast-food-style items, namely hot dogs, hamburgers, pizza, and deep-fried chicken nuggets. According to David Jacobs, a Washington, D.C., internist and specialist in clinical nutrition, "The type of food eaten in childhood is likely to form a lifelong nutritional pattern." School lunches should be a model for children, because they are in effect teaching children what is nutritionally good for them. If they learn about eating low-sugar, low-fat foods in the classroom and get just the opposite in the lunchroom, what message are the children getting?

Why do the schools serve so much junk food to our children? One important reason is that schools get foods donated by the government. These are the surplus foods that the government must buy from farmers. This requirement for using surplus foods was actually part of the Child Nutrition Act of 1946 that is the guideline for school lunches. It says that the school lunch program not only must satisfy the nutritional needs of children, but it must also aid the agriculture industry as an effective farm support program. The U.S. Department of Agriculture forgot about the first part of the guideline in favor of the second part. So whatever surplus arises—white flour, white rice, ground beef, and so on—winds up as school lunch.

If your child's school lunch fits the above description, we suggest that you send a school lunch with your child—one containing nutritious foods you know will be eaten. Preparing a bag lunch doesn't have to be a burden. Most children are satisfied with having a few favorite foods for lunch and will not demand a variety of foods. Sandwiches should be made with 100% whole-grain bread rather than "enriched" white bread with its high sugar content. Also, you can purchase 100% peanut butter—the old-fashioned kind without saturated and partially hydrogenated fats, sugars, and additives. Health food stores and supermarkets keep this type of peanut butter in stock. Wheat germ or brewer's yeast can be mixed into the peanut butter for more nutrition. Honey can be added to make the taste more appealing for children who have become accustomed to a sweetened product.

So far, you've made sure that your child has a clean mouth and a tummy full of nutritious food. Now it's time to go to the dentist!

CHAPTER 9

Going to the Dentist

It's important right from the beginning that you and your child develop a relationship with a good dentist. The first impressions about going to the dentist will stay with your child for the rest of his or her life. Choosing a good dentist means first knowing what questions to ask. When should your child's first visit be? Are X-rays necessary, and how can you (and the dentist) make them safer for your child? What's the story on tooth sealants? Are they safe and effective? To pull or not to pull (out a tooth): that is a good question. If a tooth is lost from injury, should it be replaced? You'll find the answers to these questions and more in this chapter.

According to a 1987 report by the National Center for Health Statistics, only 5% of children in the United States under age 2 had ever seen a dentist.

Getting Parents Involved

In 1986, the American Academy of Pediatric Dentistry officially recommended that parents take their children to a dental office for a first visit soon after the eruption of the first incisors, or somewhere around 12 months of age. At first, this worried dentists because they were not trained in dental school to know how to manage infants. These dentists were happy to learn that involving parents helped them handle young children. A 1-year-old sitting in a parent's lap can undergo the same mouth, head, and neck exam that can be done on a 3-year-old. Also, by starting out this way, the children got used to the dentist much more easily.

Part of the reason for having parents present has to do with legal rules. It used to be that dentists could cover the mouth of a screaming child with their hand or physically restrain the child. Now the hand over the mouth is a thing of the past, and any type of restraint requires informed consent in writing. Dentists would rather avoid these scenarios, and so many prefer to have the parent there to handle any problems. The other side of the story is that parents should not try to cater to their child's every whim about what to do in the dentist's office. There are many dentists who do not want parents in the room, and they have very good reasons.

One such dentist is Marvin Berman, D.D.S., who has been practicing pediatric dentistry for 38 years and is an associate professor at both Northwestern University and the University of Illinois dental schools. Dr. Berman has seen children of every behavior type: "Some are shy and quiet, some reluctant, while others are whiny or belligerent. There are also those who are so willful that they are almost murdering their parents in the waiting room." Dr. Berman believes that it's important to recognize each type, because each will be managed differently.

Dr. Jane Soxman, a board-certified pediatric dentist in Allison Park, Pennsylvania, and nationally known speaker and author, believes that the majority of children are very cooperative. Those children who don't behave, she says, are generally fearful. The dentist sees misbehavior as resistance, but to the child misbehavior is protection from the unknown. The dentist and his or her staff need to be trained in behavioral techniques—in how to handle young children. Many dentists don't get this training or don't want to take time for behavioral management of children, because they rarely get paid for the extra time. Pediatric dentists, however, are trained to handle frightened or misbehaving children and don't have to take extra time to do it.

Dr. Soxman says that the things children fear most are injections, choking, and drilling. The method to deal with the fears is: "tell, show, do." Here are some techniques that Dr. Soxman uses: Explain each step to the child, pat the child often on the shoulder, and ask, "How are you doing?" Tell the child how he or she can let the dentist know if something bothers them when their mouth is full—raise a hand, for example. Never use the word *hurt*. Talk about the child's favorite cartoon character: "Bugs Bunny would open his mouth wide!" During an injection, have the child raise a leg as a distraction. Let the child watch a movie using special glasses. Let the child see a brother or sister being treated. Add humor whenever possible. Morning appointments are more successful when the child and the dentist are not tired. Three weeks between appointments is recommended for a fearful child or one who requires some management. In this way, the child gets a chance to "regroup".

Sometimes it may be necessary to put off the work with a difficult child. Just watching the tooth and checking again in 3 months can often make a lot of difference in a child's maturity and ability to cope with the dental experience.

If a parent is nervous about a child's visit, she or he should be silent or wait in the reception room, says Dr. Soxman. The dentist should tell Mom or Dad how anxiety will affect the child. If the parent must leave, a good method is to leave the car keys with the child so that the child will know he or she is not abandoned and that Mom or Dad will be back.

Dr. Berman believes that the sooner you separate the child from the parent, the better. This is the view held by Dr. Mittelman and Bev Mittelman. Once a parent trusts the dentist, it is much better to have the parent wait outside—in fact, the parent should not go with the child into the dental office, because leaving them there is worse. Dr. Berman says that in his experience, children are smarter today, but a lot less well behaved than they were when he started practicing dentistry in the 1960s. Many don't get any discipline from their parents. So separating parent and child is best, according to Dr. Berman.

Before you start thinking that he is mean and nasty, let us say that Dr. Berman has a great talent with misbehaving children. He starts by showing anything that is unfamiliar (like a light or mouth mirror or probe) to the child and explaining what it is for. He will give a 2- or 3-year-old a toothbrush in a favorite color, show her where the water is, and have her brush her teeth. Then he hands her a mirror—but it's too dark to see how well her teeth were cleaned, so the dentist has a good excuse to turn on the overhead light. Each step along the way, there is explanation and motivation. Then he calls the mother or father in to see how good her child is. If a child cries for no apparent reason, Dr. Berman never says, "Shut up," "Be quiet," or "Hush." He says, "Oh, there is so much noise. You're waking my baby." He will ask the child what is the matter.

One of Dr. Berman's key rules is never, never act or react in anger. He advises: "Don't ever say, 'You bad boy,' or 'You terrible child.'" He will say to the child, "You're not being nice to me; I'm being good to you, but you're not being good to me; I hope you will be better next time." Dr. Berman will tell the parent that the child hasn't behaved well. He will never use his hand over a child's mouth.

Dr. Soxman will not do this either. She will also not sedate a child with medicine just to get the dental work done. If she has a child with many cavities and that child is completely unmanageable, she will have a dental anesthesiologist sedate the child for a brief time and only if the child is healthy. An outpatient hospital admission for general anesthesia may be necessary for some children, she believes. She would not put a child to sleep herself in the dental office. Dr. Berman also does not use sedation or nitrous oxide (see chapter X). He feels that dentists should be educators and must make a good impression on very young children. "It's not the time to knock the kid out and make him believe he is somewhere else," says Dr. Berman. He doesn't want to teach children that you use drugs at every drop of the hat—they may learn this lesson and go on to accept drug use when they are older.

Dr. Berman, who is a father of four and grandparent of five children, really believes children will behave better when parents are not in the room. He has a sign that reads "Children only—Parents by invitation." He tells parents that he likes to meet the child first and establish a good relationship. Parents who are themselves afraid of being in a dental office feel they must "protect" their child, and their attitude will create anxiety in the child. So Dr. Berman says keep out. When he and the child are having fun, he does let the parent in from behind to see what's happening. Then the parent is very content to be out in the waiting room.

While Dr. Soxman will allow parents, especially of very young children, in the dental office, she will discuss what will happen beforehand with the parent. Her rules are one parent at a time (she has had two parents fighting over what should be done for the child), very little talking, and especially not contradicting what she is telling the child. She will give the parent a job to do: pat the child, hold the hand, or help hold the mirror if the child is watching the procedure. She finds that some parents do not want to be present, so she will always ask a parent beforehand.

You can see from the above that dentists differ in their approach in handling children during dental work. Each child is different. The parents and the dentist should work out a plan for managing the child. Dentists today have become more sensitive to the various personalities and needs of children. They try to avoid causing fear in the child and have a successful visit, with all work completed. Together, parents and the dental staff can work together to make the dental experience less traumatic for the child.

According to research by the *Journal of Clinical Pediatric Dentistry,* 75% of dental professionals consider parents to be a hindrance to the behavior of preschool children in the dental office. For this reason, these offices keep parents out of the treatment room. But the study showed that there was no real difference in behavior whether the parent was with the child or not. The researchers found that most parents wished to be with their children during treatment. Only one third thought their child would behave better without them present. Some parents wanted to stay outside because they were afraid of dental work and didn't want their child to see their anxiety; in this case, the researchers believed, it might be better if they stayed outside. The researchers' conclusion was that having parents present was fine and that parents could be a valuable ally to the dentist and staff during the treatment process.

Making the Dental Visit Almost Fun

Debra Mondrow is a dental hygienist working in Mahwah, New Jersey. She makes life easy for the children who come to her for a cleaning or to see the dentist. Debra prepares each child for the experience. "Giving the child control over the situation is most important for making the visit a positive experience," says Debra. For example, a child may come in with his or her mother while the mother is getting work done. Debra will let the child have a ride in the dental chair. She will use the dental polisher on her fingernails and that of the child (if the child agrees) so that the child will know how it feels. She will sing, "This is the way we brush our teeth" while polishing the fingernails.

"Children are more likely to accept instruments in their mouth if they first touch or feel them on their hands—it's more frightening to just have something placed in the mouth without warning," says Debra. She lets the child stand up in the dental chair or sit in a parent's lap when they get work done. She will count teeth with them and tell them she will polish each tooth and give them pretty (or handsome) smiles.

Each child is different. Although Debra would rather have the parent wait outside, she will ask the child to choose between having a parent stay or sit outside. Once a child refused to come out from under a chair in the waiting room. Debra crawled under the chair with the child and talked in a whisper until she found out what was frightening him.

To make the child more comfortable, Debra will cut cotton rolls in half so that the child's mouth is not stuffed. She will crimp or fold the corners of X-ray films so that they will not dig into the child's mouth. For pain, she recommends that a children's non-aspirin-containing painkiller be given before the visit. If novocaine is used, it is in much lower amounts than adults receive. She doesn't believe that nitrous oxide (laughing gas) is safe for small children. She also doesn't believe that children under 6 years old should get X-rays routinely. "If there is a deformity of a tooth or other problem, that would be a cause for an X-ray," says Debra. "Two small bite-wing X-rays are all that's needed if a child is X-rayed—a full mouth set wouldn't be necessary until a child goes for orthodontic work."

One child had a large piece of tartar down near the gum line, but was afraid to let Debra get it out. Debra took an X-ray, showed the child where the tartar was, and explained that it would start causing tooth decay if not removed. She said it would hurt a little to get the tartar out, but the child didn't object after seeing the "whole picture."

Debra thinks sealants are good for cavity-prone children. She has seen the sealant last from when a child is 8 years old to 17 years of age. About whiteners, she says that they are too strong for young children's delicate teeth. "When it's a case of self-esteem, such as a child or teenager whose teeth are darkened from tetracycline [an antibiotic] and won't smile, then I would approve of whitening," says Debra. On the topic of fluoride, Debra says that in areas where there is no fluoride in the drinking water, fluoride treatments or supplements may be needed to prevent cavities. She says that fluoride in water or in a dietary supplement is considered systemic—it is being taken into the child's body and is much stronger (and more toxic) than getting a fluoride treatment on the outside of a tooth in the dentist's office. However, remember that all the sources of fluoride add up (see chapter 10). As a summary, Debra says, "If you remember that each child has different fears and different needs—and you treat each child as an individual—the dental experience could almost be fun for your child."

Doctors Berman and Soxman and hygienist Debra Morrow, all use much the same techinques that the Mittelmans used in their office. But the most important thing is that they use the same approach. That is, to treat a child like an adult, but not expect the child to act like one.

How to Find the Right Dentist

As a first step, you can ask your regular dentist if he or she treats children. If not, he or she can give you a referral to a dentist in your area that treats children. Asking friends or family members about their experiences with dentists can also help you find a good dentist. There's a new breed of dentist today—those who practice what is called "minimal intervention dentistry." According to Max Anderson, D.D.S., formerly of the University of Washington School of Dentistry, instead of "drill, fill, and bill," these dentists believe that the best treatment is the kind that does the least damage to the teeth. They don't believe in drilling out large areas around decay because this weakens the tooth. Each time a tooth is refilled, the crater is enlarged, making the tooth even weaker. Eventually it can lead to root canal surgery and even loss of the tooth. By doing less drilling, dentists of the new school want to stop this process before it begins. A spot of decay in a tooth doesn't always keep getting larger and larger. Sometimes it stops and the tooth may repair itself (remineralize), meaning its surface heals over. A dentist who has to drill every little spot of decay immediately is not giving this process a chance to happen. It may be better just to watch the tooth for a while. Some questions to ask a dentist to find out whether he or she is a driller or a watcher are:

1. Do you emphasize prevention? (This doesn't mean just X-rays, cleanings, and twice-a-year checkups. You want to hear that the dentist evaluates each situation, knows about mouth bacteria, and knows about dietary and lifestyle changes.)
2. Do you agree to keep old fillings in my child's teeth for as long as possible? (The dentist should agree with you.)
3. How much tooth structure do you remove around a decayed area? (You want to hear that he or she doesn't remove good tooth as well.)
4. What continuing-education courses do you and your staff take? (You want to know that the dentist stays on top of things.)

These types of questions show that you are concerned about what is done to your child. They make the dentist stop and think. Many dentists know how to work conservatively, but may not think about it until you ask. You have to be an involved parent. Speak up. Ask questions about what will be done. If you are not comfortable with what the dentist wants to do, get another opinion.

Today, it's not just the types and methods of treatment that are changing in pediatric dentistry. Over half the people in the entering classes for pediatric dentistry residency programs are women. This will lead to significant changes, which started in the year 2000. In the 1999 survey, 33% of the pediatric dentists who entered practice since 1987 were women. (Pediatric dentist looks toward next century. *Dental Products Report,* Feb. 1997)

Here are some signs that you have a good dentist:

1. While the dentist is checking the gums and teeth, he or she calls out numbers to an assistant who writes them down. These numbers are those of the teeth that need to be checked or worked on.
2. The dentist feels and looks at your child's cheeks, tongue, and the roof and floor of the mouth at least once a year. This is done to see if there are signs of health problems such as sores or infections.
3. The dentist takes X-rays of the entire mouth every 3 or 4 years. This is done to check for cavities and also to see the health of the jawbone and other structures supporting the teeth.
4. The dentist tries to keep pain to a minimum. Advances in pain management such as superfast drills and no-needle painkillers mean that dental work doesn't have to hurt.
5. He or she takes time to explain what is going on in your child's mouth and what will be done. Also, at each visit the dentist or a hygienist should discuss proper diet, brushing, and flossing.

What Is Preventive Dentistry?

A pediatric dentist, one that specializes in treating children, should practice preventive dentistry. According to the AAPD, preventive dentistry for children includes:

• Watching your child's dental development and explaining it to you

- Stressing the importance of brushing and flossing and making sure that you and your child know to do these things correctly
- Being aware of oral habits such as thumb sucking and recommending solutions to problems
- Understanding the proper use of orthodontics (teeth straightening)
- Getting parents involved in their child's dental health practices (like brushing and flossing)
- Recommending a proper diet
- Understanding the pros and cons of sealants
- Explaining sports safety and what to do if a tooth is knocked out or injured

According to the AAPD, "Preventive dentistry means a healthy smile for your child. Children with healthy mouths chew more easily and gain more nutrients from the foods they eat. They learn to speak more quickly and clearly. They have a better chance of general health, because disease in the mouth can endanger the rest of the body. A healthy mouth is more attractive, giving children confidence in their appearance. Finally, preventive dentistry means less extensive, and less expensive, treatment for your child."

Children's or pediatric dentistry has improved over the last 15 years. It has gone from just restoring caries to stopping them from forming in the first place. Besides preventive care, infant dental care, and behavioral techniques such as having parents present, your child will benefit from other changes. Dentists are now more concerned about the safety and biohazards of mercury in amalgam fillings. This concern and wanting to improve the look of dental work have created an interest in developing materials that are safer as well as more pleasing to look at. The names are technical, but you can ask your dentist about them: resin-modified glass ionomer cements, gallium-based alloys, hybrid composite resins, and compomers. The glass ionomer so far seems to last the longest. Instead of using stainless steel crowns (caps) for baby teeth, there are now crowns just as strong, with natural-looking facings.

"In the past ten years, the major development [in pediatric dentistry] has been a change in emphasis to the prevention of disease rather than the repair of its damages." (Dr. Theodore Croll, Bucks County, Pennsylvania, pediatric dentist)

The First Dental Visit

Your child's first visit to the dental office should be around his or her first birthday, but could be as early as you'd like (as soon as the first tooth erupts or even sooner). In 1997, the general recommendation was to wait no later than age 2. Now, it is recommended that the first visit be within 6 months of the first primary tooth's eruption and no later than age 1.

If you notice a cavity, or if a tooth is injured, you should see a dentist immediately. The earlier you begin, the better chance your dentist has to prevent problems. Note that baby teeth are small and decay can quickly reach the nerve and kill the tooth. Here are some do's and don'ts.

Do:

- Take a tour of the dental office before an actual visit. Make it a casual, friendly get-acquainted visit. Don't wait until your child is in pain to see the dentist. If your child is frightened or uncomfortable, make more than one (short) visit to build trust in the dentist and the dental office.
- Make an appointment for a visual check of your child's teeth. Make the appointment early in the day, when he or she will be alert and not cranky from needing a nap.
- Have a discussion with your dental hygienist or dentist about oral health care for your child.
- Familiarize your children with the dental office. Consider taking them along when you or a sibling has a dental appointment. You may want to have your child sit in your lap while you are in the dental chair.

Don't:

- Wait for an emergency for the first visit.
- Overprepare your children for dental visits; too much emphasis may make them afraid.
- Use phrases like "It won't hurt much" or "It won't be too bad." Such phrases do not soothe; they only create anxiety.

Some dental offices provide a free first dental visit for children under the age of 3. Call your dental office to find out if they are participating in such a program.

Make sure that your child does not have an empty stomach when you go to the dentist. Giving local anesthetic to a child (or to anyone) with low blood sugar (due to not eating) causes a lot of stress for both child and dentist. Your child will be a lot less cooperative. The dentist should ask what your child had last to eat and when. A meal high in carbohydrates, especially refined sugars, can put your child on an emotional roller coaster for the rest of the day. It's important that your child have a high-protein breakfast (with eggs, cheese, meat, or tofu) or other meal before coming to the dentist whether or not an anesthetic will be given.

What to Expect During the First Visit

If your child is ready, the first dental examination should last between 15 and 30 minutes and may include the following:

1. The dentist will do a gentle but thorough examination of the teeth, jaw, bite, gums, and oral tissues.
2. If needed, there will be a gentle cleaning, which includes polishing teeth and removing any plaque, tartar buildup, or stains.
3. X-rays may be taken (see protection suggestions on page 236).
4. There should be a demonstration on proper home cleaning of your child's teeth.
5. The dentist should be able to answer any questions you have and try to make you and your child feel comfortable throughout the visit.

6. The entire dental team should provide a relaxed, nonthreatening environment for your child.

Latex allergies. From 1% to 6% of people are allergic to natural rubber latex. This material is heavily used in dental and medical offices and hospitals. In the dentist's office, latex rubber gloves are used. The rubber dams (plugs) used to hold open the mouth are often made of latex rubber. Tubing, rubber bands, and even the backing on floor mats may contain latex. Symptoms of latex allergy are swelling of the area that comes in contact with the latex, such as the lips and cheeks. People who are very sensitive can have a reaction when the dentist snaps off the latex rubber gloves and the powder gets into the air around the patient. Although dentists and other health professionals are becoming aware of this problem, it's a good idea to ask your dentist whether he or she uses latex products, especially if you believe your child may be sensitive to latex.

The next visit after the first one should be in 6 months. Some dentists may want to see your child every 3 months when the child is very young to build up his or her confidence.

Which Teeth Come In When?

Teeth start forming in your baby's jaws during your 5th month of pregnancy (a good reason to have good nourishment during pregnancy). The crowns that form are the crowns of the first set of 20 "milk," "baby," or as they are also called, deciduous teeth. At birth, these 20 teeth are in the jaws waiting to erupt. Some babies are born with 1 or 2 teeth already cut and in sight. This is usually hereditary. These early teeth are usually the 2 lower front teeth (incisors or cutters). These teeth may cause problems nursing, but it is not a good idea to remove them. Doing so may affect the formation of the jaws and cause later crowding or spacing of the first and second set of teeth and future orthodontist visits to straighten teeth.

Children will cut their first teeth at different times. Just when varies from child to child and from family to family, but it does follow a fairly normal pattern. The 2 lower front center teeth (incisors) are usually the first to appear, at about 6 or 7 months. The upper front centrals, or incisors, usually appear from 9 months to 1 year. After that the rest of the 20 baby teeth erupt and become visible by the age of 2 or 3 years. These teeth will be what your child eats with until the first permanent teeth erupt—the first molars—at about age 6. The first molars begin the second set of permanent teeth that will eventually number 32. These teeth are important because they help shape the lower part of your child's face. They also affect the position and health of the other permanent teeth that will soon follow.

> Six is the magic number in timing when teeth cut. Just about the 6th month of pregnancy, the tips of the crowns of the baby teeth form. About 6 months after birth, these first teeth will erupt above the gum line. At about 6 years of age children start to cut the permanent teeth with the appearance of the first molars. Six years later at about age 12, the second molars come in behind the first molars. Also at this age children lose the last of the baby teeth. The other permanent teeth erupt, for a total of 28. Then, about 6 years later, at the age of 18 or so, the last 4 teeth back in the jaws erupt. These are the third molars, or wisdom teeth. They sometimes remain buried, wedged under the 12-year molars, or impacted, causing great discomfort. All this timing, remember, can vary from one child to another by a few weeks or months, and even a year or two.

In some cases, a tooth may have trouble trying to cut through the gum, and the dentist will have to cut or lance the gums. When teeth are cutting you may also see a large to medium-large purplish colored, round vesicle or lump on your child's gums. This is usually due to a slowly erupting tooth. If it has not broken and disappeared within 48 hours, show it to your dentist.

Don't worry about teeth being a little late to come in. The slower and later that teeth erupt, the stronger they will usually be. The faster and earlier, the weaker these teeth will be. This is because if teeth form too fast, there is less time for them to get fully calcified. Teeth which erupt later than normal are practically always strong, hard, and well formed. Early-erupting teeth almost always develop more flaws and need more careful checking and more dental attention. Although just when the teeth will come up has to do with heredity, malnutrition or illness can affect the timing.

The primary (or baby) teeth are important. You can't just forget about them because a second set is on the way. Hear what Dr. Terry Gillespie a dentist in Red Oak, Iowa, has to say: "The primary teeth properly maintained form holding pillars so the jaw can develop correctly and the permanent teeth can assume their proper place in the mouth. The primary teeth influence the final position of the permanent teeth. If a primary molar is lost prematurely and steps are not taken to maintain space, a dental tragedy can occur." Don't think that it's only a back tooth and doesn't need to be fixed. All the primary teeth have important jobs to do, and some of them have to last for 10 to 12 years. These early teeth help in the development of the face and jaws, affecting the growth, height, and shape of the face. Teeth are an important part of your child's appearance and sense of self-worth.

In the case above when a tooth is missing, the bite will collapse and teeth will shift. This allows food to be entrapped, encourages plaque growth and invites decay. But it does more. With an irregular bite, the child's jaw grinds and clenches. Note that this also happens to many children as primary teeth are lost when the permanent teeth come in. It can lead to flare-up of the eustachian tubes of the middle ear, which can become infected. Many children are put on repeated courses of antibiotics when this happens. We know that this can cause many health problems over a period of time and should be kept to an absolute minimum. Prompt bite correction could alleviate much of the problem.

According to Stephen J. Moss, D.D.S., presently professor emeritus at New York University College of Dentistry (see chapter 4), some missing teeth don't have to be replaced. For those in the upper front region, spaces don't close up. But in the back of the mouth, loss of a tooth before its time may mean trouble. "Teeth don't know where they are going; if they did, we wouldn't have coined the word *malocclusion,* and orthodontists would have to find some other specialty to practice." Dr. Moss says that the back primary teeth will be in the mouth until the child is 11 or 12 years of age. If these teeth are carrying dental disease (caries) they will pass it right along to the new permanent teeth. If a primary tooth becomes infected and abscessed at the root, the infection may damage the underlying permanent tooth.

Root canal treatment (also called pulp therapy) is being done on primary teeth so that the tooth will remain in place as a natural space retainer for permanent teeth. Even if the treatment will be needed for only a few months until the permanent tooth comes in, it is worth doing it to prevent future, costly procedures. Some of the symptoms that a tooth may need root canal work are pain that comes and goes when the child is eating hot or cold food or sweets and stops when not eating these things. Without treatment at this stage, pain may become intense and last longer. If it worsens it can keep the child awake at night and painkillers (such as Tylenol) may not work. So to spare your child misery and the need for future uncomfortable and expensive orthodontic work, make sure your child's primary teeth are well cared for.

X-rays: What the Dentist Is Looking For

Tooth decay can proceed rapidly in children, and most dentists believe that it is important to detect a cavity as soon as possible. They will therefore take X-rays in order to see cavities early. Cavities still too small to be seen by the naked eye will show up on an X-ray. Also, decay spots between the teeth, where a mirror can't reach, can be found by X-ray. The dentist can also see what's under your child's gums if he thinks there is a problem. Extra teeth or missing teeth in the permanent set which are still buried in the jaw can be seen with a X-ray. The dentist needs this information in order to decide whether to keep or remove teeth. But taking X-rays is not without risk.

How to Make Taking X-rays Safer for Your Child

All X-rays put the cells of the body at risk for damage. A responsible dentist will use X-rays as little as possible. One type of X-ray that is safer for your child is called digital or filmless radiography. Traditional X-rays are done with X-ray film that is developed. This new type of X-ray cuts patients' radiation exposure by up to 90% from that of film-based X-rays. The X-ray can be shown on a computer monitor (screen) and enlarged and shown in color. This helps you to better understand what is going on in your child's mouth. Many dentists don't use this type.

While dentists will use lead aprons when taking X-rays, there are other ways to protect your child. Some dentists will use a thyroid shield that covers the front of the neck. The thyroid is a very important gland and should be protected.

What About Sealants?

Sealants have been available for almost 30 years, yet the idea is still new to many dentists and patients, and the need is not well understood. Tooth decay starts in childhood because children are especially vulnerable to it. They do not have their resistance built up, and most of the new permanent molar teeth have tiny open holes in the enamel surface. Enamel is like skin; it is supposed to protect the underlying dentin from bacteria and wear. Unfortunately, the grooves in the center of many teeth have flaws, which allow the decay to easily penetrate the tooth's protective layer. Once inside the hard enamel, decay will mushroom out into the dentin and destroy large amounts of tooth in just a few months. The best thing to do is repair the tiny flaws in the grooves in the center of many teeth with a bonded sealant before decay starts.

Sealants are plastic films painted onto the chewing surfaces of teeth to protect them from decay. Once the tooth surface is properly cleaned, a thin sealer is applied which flows into the porosity (holes) of the enamel and seals out the decay germs. This painless procedure does not require any shots or drilling. The sealants can be a tremendous cost savings to the consumer. As long as the tooth is sealed, there is 100% protection from decay on the biting surface. Sealants wear out, however, and should be replaced as needed until about age 25. By that time, the cavity-prone years are over, and there is no further benefit from sealants with the possible exception of the wisdom teeth (18-year molars).

Sealants can actually stop decay. About 80% of the decay in children's permanent teeth is located in the vulnerable grooves. New permanent molars come in at ages 6, 12, and 18. These years are the critical ones since the sealants should be applied before decay begins. However, research has shown that if a tiny amount of decay has already begun, the sealant will actually stop it.

Decay must have contact with the oral cavity; otherwise it cannot proceed. Apparently, if a few decay germs are left under the sealant they are entombed until the sealant is lost. If, on the other hand, a substantial amount of decay has already begun, then a combination sealant and restoration (filling) is indicated.

No Need to Drill Away Good Teeth

In the past, when a pinhead-sized cavity was found, dentists were taught to place a large pea-sized lump of mercury/silver in an oversized preparation. In order to do that, they drilled away about one third of the middle of the tooth. They didn't realize that excess drilling weakens the tooth 75% and often leads to broken and dead teeth (which mean root canals and crowns) later in life. With the sealant/filling there is no need to drill away any good tooth. If a pinhead-sized cavity has already begun, then a pinhead-sized filling should be placed in the area of decay and a sealant applied to the rest of the surface of the tooth.

When you go to the dentist, choose sealants for your children, rather than accept the mercury-leaking fillings or cancer-producing fluoride for your children or yourself. They are environmental blunders left over from the last century and have no place in a health-conscious world of today. Raise your children and grandchildren to be free from decay by following the advice in this book, so they never have to worry about the tooth decay damage and toxic problems of the past.

Some sealants contain fluoride (see chapter 10). No one knows exactly how much fluoride is released and what effect this toxic time-release poison will have on the child's brain, bones, kidneys, immune system, and other organs. While sealants are recommended for all permanent molars, time-release fluoride is unnecessary. There are many brands of sealants that work well and do not release any fluoride.

Some dentists believe that sealants should be used only if the child is at high risk of dental caries. Sealant treatment does not mean that regular brushing and flossing, along with proper diet, are no longer needed. Although their use doubled between 1987 and 1994, population-wide use of dental sealants remains low. The National Health and Nutrition Examination Survey found sealants on the primary teeth of less than 2% of children, and on the permanent teeth of 19% of children and adolescents.

There is controversy as to whether sealant material releases chemicals that could be harmful. One study found that a chemical, bisphenol-A (BPA), was released from dental sealants one hour after putting the sealants on teeth. This chemical has estrogenlike properties. The researchers noted that it wasn't yet known what levels of this chemical could be harmful. However, estrogen-like chemicals are known to interfere with growth and development and in some cases increase the risk of breast cancer. However, this study used high heat and strong acid or alkaline solutions to soak the dental material containing the sealants. It may be that only under such conditions, which wouldn't be found in the mouth, would there be release of bisphenol-A. Another study that used milder conditions didn't find any release of the chemical .

The problem of these chemicals being released from sealant is well recognized. There are some steps to take that can keep exposure to the sealant chemicals to a minimum. If the dentist follows the proper safety precautions, any risk from the sealant will be decreased. The resin in the sealant is the culprit. The dentist must clean off excess uncured resin before the child leaves the dental chair. Then the dentist should polish down the surface with water and lavage (wash) the whole working area, using a rubber dam wherever possible, thus minimizing the dose of chemicals from sealant applications.

Also, make sure that the dentist doesn't use sealant that contains time-release fluoride in the sealant (or in the filling material). You have the right to insist on a no-fluoride product. See chapter 10 about the details of fluoride. If the dentist is a firm believer in fluoride and refuses to leave it out, you may want to take your business elsewhere. You should discuss these issues with the dentist before you show up for an appointment with your child.

The addition of fluoride to filling materials is a new cause for concern. Dentists have in the past (and some still today) used the following toxic or caustic compounds: formaldehyde, nickel, silver, mercury, fluoride, copper, zinc, and tin, and even very small quantities of degraded uranium (radioactive) in filling material. Hopefully, today's dentists are moving toward more natural methods of dental care.

How do you avoid or minimize some of the dangers your child faces? The ideal action to take is to give your child a really healthy diet from the time you are carrying the child—low sugar, lots of vegetables (see chapter 7)—in order to prevent the need for sealants. However, if a child is cavity-prone, it would make better sense to use sealants to prevent decay rather than repair decay once it has occurred. Repair is a less satisfactory solution, and it also may involve chemicals such as mercury.

> In one study, sealants were completely intact on 28% of sealed teeth 15 years later. In 35% of the teeth, the sealant was partially intact. Dentists doing the study calculated that during 15 years an unsealed tooth surface was 7.5 times more likely to decay than one that was sealed. If lost sealants are replaced as needed, prevention of cavities on sealed surfaces could reach 100%.

To Bleach or Not to Bleach?

Many people want white teeth—for themselves and for their children as well. One problem with bleaching teeth, however, is that it weakens the enamel. Although tooth color is mostly hereditary, there are substances that can discolor teeth. Giving the antibiotic tetracycline to young children can cause permanent discoloration of the teeth. Adolescent children given long-term treatment with tetracycline for acne also get discoloration. Excess fluoride can also cause dark spots on the teeth (see chapter 10). Tooth whiteners really defeat the purpose they are intended for. They may whiten teeth. However, they also weaken enamel at the same time. We mentioned before that soda pop can weaken teeth by causing loss of calcium from the bone that holds our teeth in the jaw. Add soda pop to already weakened enamel (from whiteners), and there may be even more damage. Coloring dyes in the acidic soda pop may sink into the weakened tooth enamel, discoloring the teeth. Again, good nutrition starting from before conception and avoiding substances that can cause discoloration of teeth are the better choice.

According to ADA spokesperson Matthew Messina, D.D.S., the materials in over-the-counter bleaching kits have not yet received FDA approval and do not carry the American Dental Association Seal of Acceptance. "In general, we've found that these products don't work all that well and carry a pretty high risk of gum irritation."

Tooth Trauma: What to Do

It's important to know what to do if an injury causes damage or loss of your child's tooth. If your child falls or gets hit in the mouth, and there is mild bleeding from the gums and slightly loose teeth, healing usually happens within 3 days. Sucking on ice may ease the pain. If the tooth is very loose (can move more than one eighth of an inch) or is painful, becomes discolored, or sensitive to cold or heat, call your dentist. What should you do if a primary (baby) tooth gets knocked out or is broken, cracked, or pushed out of line? Consult your dentist immediately. In the months immediately after a tooth is lost, there is the most amount of movement of other teeth into the empty space. This will affect how the permanent teeth come in. Your dentist may recommend a space maintainer, especially if a primary second molar is lost, because this tooth is a key to the normal development of the permanent teeth. A maintainer is a metal or plastic appliance that holds the space open until the permanent tooth comes in.

If a permanent tooth gets knocked out, save it. The biggest threats to the free tooth are dehydration and infection. The tooth should be held by the crown (top), gently washed (not scrubbed), and placed back in the mouth in position. Do not touch the root at all if possible. Tell your child to bite down on a wad of gauze or cloth until you get to the dentist's office (or hospital emergency room if you can't get to a dentist). If you are worried about doing this, the tooth should be placed immediately in liquid or in a clean, wet cloth, or better still, in a glass or plastic container holding the liquid. Water is not the best liquid to use as it may be absorbed too fast into the root and the root cells may burst. This will kill the tooth and make implantation unlikely. The only thing worse is to keep the tooth dry. You can soak the tooth in milk (skim or low-fat is better than whole milk), but the important thing is to get the tooth into liquid quickly. Even contact-lens wetting solution can be used if nothing else is available. Try to get to the dentist within 30 minutes if possible. It is a good idea to talk to your dentist *before* something like this happens and to work out a plan of what to do. He or she should have a tooth "first aid kit" ready for such an emergency.

The dentist may be able to replant the tooth and apply a splint that will keep it in position until it has reattached itself to the jaw and is able to function normally. In some cases the dentist will place the teeth in special solutions that will "revive" the tooth cells. Broken teeth can often be repaired with excellent materials your dentist has available.

After the dentist treats your child, he or she may have pain. You can help reduce the pain with clove oil, an old-time herbal remedy still used in dentists' offices today. It relieves pain and disinfects the area around the hurt tooth. A child's gums are sensitive, so dilute one to two drops of clove oil in a teaspoon of vegetable oil. Moisten a cotton swab with the mixture and apply directly to the injured area. It can be applied again in a half hour, using a fresh cotton swab.

How can you guard against tooth injuries? If your child plays contact sports like football or soccer, make sure he or she wears a mouth protector. You can buy one or your dentist can make a custom-fitted guard. Don't let your child chew ice. While it may seem like fun, it can be disaster for the teeth. The crunching and cracking may not be just the ice—it may be the teeth! Here's what happens: ice is very cold and teeth are much warmer. When the ice cube is in the mouth, the cold causes the fibers in the tooth's enamel to shrink. Then, when your child finishes the cube, the tooth warms up and expands again. Doing this over and over can make the tooth enamel brittle. Finally, an ice cube cracks the tooth—maybe even deeply enough to expose the nerve. Usually, the ice may cause a small crack that is not noticed. But it may develop into a more serious fracture later. Many times these cracks cannot be seen when looking at the tooth, and X-rays cannot always pick them up. There may be discomfort in the tooth and the reason may not be found. So don't let your child chew ice.

Some more advice: Don't let your child chew on pencils or pens. This can cause tiny stress fractures in the teeth, setting the stage for future problems. Don't let your child use toothpicks. Digging around the base of a tooth can loosen the connective tissue that holds the tooth in place. It can also dislodge a filling, embed a splinter in the gums, or, most dangerous of all, be swallowed.

How You Can Help Your Child Have a Positive Attitude About Dental Visits

Although dentists have lots of ways to prevent pain, it is the fear and apprehension that will make the experience feel worse than it is. So it's important to prepare your child mentally for a trip to the dentist. Talk about going to the dentist in a positive, matter-of-fact way. Tell your child that the dentist is a friendly person who will help keep his or her teeth healthy. Never allow your child to overhear unpleasant stories of dental work. Many parents have their own fears of going to the dentist. They may have been held in the dentist's chair as children, or ignored when they were experiencing pain. You don't want to transmit these fears to your child. Developing a friendly relationship between your child and the dental staff will help prevent the fear that makes a child not want to go to a dentist (and in the future, as an adult, to postpone dental work). Your own attitude is very important: you set the example that will shape your child's feelings about dental care for years to come. A mother's anxiety is the biggest factor affecting a child's first visit to the dentist. "Her apprehension is transmitted to the child," says Dr. Marvin Berman, a Chicago specialist in children's dentistry. "She will remember certain aspects of her own visit to the dentist and transmit these fears." An example of anxiety, said Berman, is the mother who says, "Don't worry" to a child entering the dental office. "She doesn't say that to the child when taking him to fit a pair of shoes," he pointed out. "The child wonders what she meant by 'Don't worry.' "

The majority of children are at least anxious when going to the dentist for the first time. A dentist that uses the right techniques can change a terrified child into a cooperative patient—a child who will leave the office with a smile on his or her face. According to James F. Thompson, a dentist in Los Altos, California, the first thing a dentist must do is convince the child of his honesty. Children are smart and not easily fooled. If the dentist makes a promise, it must be kept. If the dentist tells the child that he will count teeth, then it must happen. "The dentist has to prove that he can be trusted to do exactly what he says he is going to do—no more, no less," says Dr. Thompson.

Over the years, the Mittelmans have developed some methods that will help keep you and your child more comfortable during dental visits. Make sure your child is not hungry when he or she gets to the dental office. Low blood sugar can cause a child (or an adult) to become irritable and more sensitive to sensations associated with treatment. It is especially bad to give a local anesthetic injection to someone with low blood sugar—it can cause shakiness and dizziness. Low blood sugar starts after about 4 hours without food, possibly in less time in an active child. So at least an hour before the visit, give your child a light meal or snack—one that is not high in refined sugars (see chapter 7). Some dentists serve patients a protein drink when they come in for treatment. This is a sound kindness. We are totally against any beverages containing caffeine, such as soda or hot cocoa. The caffeine will first raise blood sugar levels, but shortly will drop them even lower than before in some cases. This results in low energy, fatigue, and irritability. Nuts or a slice of cheese is a good snack. There are some calming methods that we have learned from John Diamond, M.D., a psychiatrist who practices holistic healing. Some of them can be used with children:

- Tell your child to clasp hands on his or her belly. This is much more calming than putting arms on the armrest.
- Use Rescue Remedy, a combination of Bach Flower Essences (discussed later in this chapter). Put a drop or two in the mouth before treatment. We kept a dropper bottle of Rescue

Remedy at each dental chair. You can get it at many health food stores.

- Let your child wear a stereo with earphones with favorite music playing on it.
- Tell your child not to stare into the fluorescent lights above.
- If your dentist has not already done so, have him explain just what will be done to the child. Fear of the unknown is one of the worst fears.

Your Child and Dental Pain

How do you explain to a child that something that hurts is good for him or her? Pain and the fear of pain are the main reasons why adult patients try to avoid or do avoid dental care. Scientists know that pain in the face and teeth can cause exaggerated responses: the crying or yelling can be louder than expected. This is because the face and teeth are very important to how we think about ourselves. We are more emotional about what happens in this area. One of the reasons for using good pain relief procedures is that the longer the pain goes on, the more fear and anxiety the child feels. This leads to a stronger pain feeling. Also, each person responds differently to pain. In a familiar surrounding or with people your child knows, he or she may feel less pain. A good dentist takes on the responsibility of controlling pain and we will discuss some natural remedies for pain below.

A report presented at the Annual Meeting of the Pediatric Academic Societies, May 4, 1999, found that there are seven drug-free techniques for relieving pain in children: biofeedback, massage, relaxation therapy, hypnosis, guided imagery, meditation, and acupuncture.

Good and Not-So-Good Ways to Deal With Pain

Managing dental pain in children is a particularly challenging task. Young children usually cannot express themselves well when something hurts. If their pain is not prevented or controlled, going to the dentist will become a frightening experience—one that the child will always want to avoid. While local anesthetics (injections) and nitrous oxide (laughing gas) can alleviate pain, these drugs have side effects. Detoxification systems in children don't work as well as those for adults, so drugs have a worse effect on them. There are however, natural alternatives to dental drugs. These natural remedies can help children both psychologically and physically prepare for and tolerate dental pain.

For children, and even for adults, the fear of pain is the main reason for delaying or avoiding a visit to the dentist. If this fear can be eliminated or even reduced, the pain itself will decrease. Our brains have their own system for dealing with pain. The brain can make natural painkillers called endorphins. When we are afraid or anxious, however, we don't make these natural painkillers as well as we can when we are calm. Other chemical changes resulting from fear can also decrease the painkilling effects of drugs given for pain. So controlling pain starts long before a child sits in the dental chair.

According to Stanton Wolfe, a dentist and former lecturer at Yale University Medical Center, the mental part of pain control starts with the receptionist in the dentist's office. Everybody who works in the dental office, according to Dr. Wolfe, should show that they are caring. There are many ways to calm an anxious patient, starting with simple breathing exercises and music or TV. Some dentists will give a child a mirror and explain what is being done, or will have headsets with children's stories or music. Using an egg timer to show the child that the procedure will take only 5 minutes makes it easier for the child to understand compared with just telling how long it will be.

Nitrous Oxide Is No Laughing Matter

Nitrous oxide, also called "laughing gas" or "sweet air," is neither funny nor sweet. Its ability to relax and relieve anxiety comes with side effects that can harm patients and dental staff as well. About 85% of pediatric dentists and 50% of general practitioners use nitrous oxide in their practices. Among the dangers of nitrous oxide (abbreviated as N_2O) is hypoxia, which means not enough oxygen in the blood. The N_2O is given together with oxygen. If the machine is not adjusted properly, all N_2O can be coming out and no oxygen. This can cause unconsciousness or even death if it goes unnoticed.

Nutrient deficiencies can affect the response to N_2O. In one study five patients developed degeneration of the spinal cord after getting N_2O. What the dentists didn't know was that the patients were deficient in vitamin B_{12}, which made them very sensitive to N_2O. The gas causes a reaction in the body that makes the vitamin B_{12} inactive. It also interferes with levels of folic acid (the B vitamin) and causes deficiencies of both B_{12} and folic acid. The nerves in the spinal cord (and elsewhere in the body) need B_{12} to function normally. People who will be taking nitrous oxide for several hours should be supplemented with both B_{12} and folate. Dentists should make sure that their patients don't have B_{12} deficiency before giving N_2O.

As we mentioned in chapter 2, N_2O can cause fertility problems in female and male dental staff. While the gas doesn't affect patients (as far as researchers know), long-term, low-level exposure of women working in dental offices can affect the staff. Almost 25 years ago, studies showed that N_2O caused spontaneous abortions to increase 2.3 times for female dental assistants and 1.5 times for unexposed wives of male dentists. More recent studies showed increased risk of spontaneous abortion in women who worked with N_2O for 3 or more hours a week in offices not using scavenging equipment that removes the N_2O gas from the air in the office. Not all dentists use the scavenging equipment either. A 1991 American Dental Association Survey of Dental Practice found that 58% of general and specialty dentists used N_2O, but one third lacked scavenging equipment.[2] Even though there is equipment that is said to be "safe and effective" in removing N_2O, not all of the machines work properly.

Again, the harmful effect of N_2O on vitamin B_{12} explains the infertility. Vitamin B_{12} is needed to make an enzyme (methionine synthetase) that is necessary for ovulation and early development of the fertilized egg. N_2O also interferes with the release of hormones from the brain that are necessary for fertility. Giving vitamin B_{12} supplements to dental staff may help protect them from the hazards of N_2O.

Does Your Dentist Know?

The Centers for Disease Control's National Institute for Occupational Safety and Health (NIOSH) issues alerts on workplace hazards that have caused death, serious injury, or illness to workers. One such alert is the Request for Assistance in Controlling Exposures to Nitrous Oxide During Anesthetic Administration. It says that workers exposed to nitrous oxide may have problems with fertility and decreases in mental performance, vision and hearing, and problems with skills using their hands. This alert tells workers how to prevent or substantially reduce exposure to nitrous oxide on the job. Dentists concerned about the safety of their staff will follow the NIOSH rules.

Hazards of general anesthesia

Children are usually given an injection of lidocaine and epinephrine for pain. The epinephrine is added so that the lidocaine doesn't get washed away by the blood. It does this by constricting blood vessels in the area of the injection. This constriction can affect your child's response to other medications he or she may be taking. Epinephrine should not be given to an asthmatic child who is taking inhalant medicine such as albuterol (Proventil or Ventolin). Doing so can cause heart palpitations, abnormal heart rhythms, rapid heartbeat, or elevated blood pressure. Your child's response to these drugs also depends on body weight. If a child is thin, lidocaine and epinephrine have a much greater effect because thin children have less blood than heavier children, so the drug is more concentrated.

Vitamin C is very good for you, but there is one time when you shouldn't take it. Because the vitamin is such a good detoxifier of chemicals and drugs, it will counteract the effect of dental local anesthesia. If taken before going to the dentist in doses of 500 milligrams or more, the painkiller may take longer to work, it may last for a shorter time, and it may not relieve the pain as well. The dentist will either have to wait until the vitamin C wears off or give more anesthetic. So save your vitamin C for *after* the dental appointment. It can help the numbing effect of the anesthetic wear off more quickly and help get rid of that "fat lip" feeling.

Dentists may also give sedation to children, sometimes by the intravenous (IV) method. According to Dr. Jane Soxman, mistakes have been made in giving drugs and deaths have resulted in dental offices. Some of these mistakes and deaths were caused by errors that the dental staff made and the rest by not knowing that some children had undiagnosed medical conditions. Dr. Soxman says that if the dentist is not skilled in starting an intravenous line, prescribing and injecting the right medications, interpreting a heart monitor, and putting in an endotracheal (breathing) tube, IV or deep sedation should not be done in a private office without the presence of a dental anesthesiologist. Respiratory function is probably the greatest concern as many of the drugs used to sedate depress (slow) breathing.

Not as much research has been done to investigate the safety and effectiveness of drugs for children as has been done for adults. The dentist should keep the following in mind when deciding on dosages of sedative dental drugs for children:

1. Proper drug dosages are based on body weight; a younger child usually should be given a smaller amount.
2. If a child is anxious, a larger dose will be needed to work.
3. The dentist should use the smallest effective dose.
4. A more active child will need a larger dose, because the drug will be metabolized (broken down and cleared from the body) more quickly.
5. Food in the stomach will change how fast the drug takes effect; usually the effect will be stronger on an empty stomach. Note, however, that not eating before going to the dentist can cause other problems (see below).
6. More sedative may be needed in the morning or just after a nap, when the child is less tired and more active.

When oral medication is given for pain (acetaminophen or ibuprofen), the child should take it in the office, not at home. In case the medicine makes the child throw up, the dentist should be there to make sure that the child doesn't aspirate (inhale) vomit into his or her lungs, causing pneumonia. The dentist should make sure that there is no congestion or blockage from mucus due to allergies or infection before giving sedation. A clear nose and throat will prevent breathing difficulty when the child is sedated. Some dentists use chest restraints to hold children in the chair (a pedo wrap). These should not be so tight that the child can't move his or her chest to breathe.

Most important, the dentist should understand what happens when two or more drugs are combined. Giving a combination of drugs can make sedation stronger. The American Academy of Pediatric Dentistry has rules for sedating children. A pulse oximeter to measure the amount of oxygen in the blood should be used, as well as a stethoscope and heart monitor. The dentist and his staff should know CPR and have a written list of what to do in an emergency posted in the dental room where the work is done. There is no way to tell (unless it has happened before) whether a child will have a bad reaction to a drug, so they must be prepared. If all this sounds terrible to you, imagine how it is for your child. This is why natural methods should be tried before resorting to such drastic measures.

On January 20, 1999, the CBS TV newsmagazine *60 Minutes II* did a show on dental anesthesia deaths in children. There was *no* public reaction to the show. The Dental Society of the State of New York and the American Dental Association did not get any inquiries from concerned parents in the weeks immediately following the broadcast. No other TV shows or newspapers did any follow-up on the report.

The Dental Society of the State of New York recommends the following steps to help protect the health and safety of your child (and anyone who goes to the dentist).

Tell your dentist about:

- Changes in your child's health since the last visit
- All drugs and medicines your child takes
- Your child's illnesses or health conditions
- Your child's allergies and reactions to medications

Some drugs should not be taken if a child or adult has liver or kidney problems.

Calming Techniques and
Natural Remedies for Pain

Because of the above problems that come with the use of dental drugs, we would like to suggest that other methods be tried. Homeopathy, Bach Flower Remedies, and stress-reducing methods may make your child comfortable enough so that he or she can do without the drugs or at least need lower doses of them.

> When we become dental patients, we try to be cooperative, try to make it possible for the dentist to do his procedure with as little stress as possible. Yes, dentists pick up tension from their patients. When we are relaxed, our dentist becomes more relaxed. Who wants to be treated by an uptight dentist?

Homeopathy

About 200 years ago, Dr. Samuel Hahnemann, a German physician, was trying to discover how medicines work. Because he wanted to avoid the side effects common with the highly toxic drugs used at that time, he used small amounts of natural active substances (plant, animal, or mineral sources). After much testing (some of it on himself) he developed what is called the Law of Similars. He found that a sick person could be helped by giving tiny amounts of substances that, in a healthy person, would give the same symptoms as the sick person had. The smaller the doses, the better the patients responded. Hahnemann found this was true for every remedy he tested. There now are nearly 2,000 remedies used to treat most common conditions like allergy, colds, flu, bruises, and dental pain. Dr. Hahnemann's belief was that the remedies act to stimulate the body's natural healing processes. They do not merely suppress or control symptoms. Since there is no "drug" effect, there are no real side effects. The remedies are nontoxic and cannot cause any actual damage.

According to *The New England Journal of Medicine* (1993), approximately 2.5 million Americans, 1% of the U.S. population, used homeopathy in 1990—an indication that it has become a growing part of American health care. And because it has no side effects, homeopathy is truly a safer medicine!

No one knows exactly how a homeopathic remedy works, only that it does work. Of course, no one knows exactly how an aspirin works, either. Although most doctors and dentists are skeptical that homeopathy really works, a growing number of conventional health professionals are finding that it has a place in modern medical treatment. According to Wayne B. Jonas, M.D., former director, National Institutes of Health Office of Complementary and Alternative Medicine, doctors need to practice what is called "evidence-based medicine." This means that the doctor must look at what is actually happening in the real world. If patients are getting better, then the therapy is useful, whether it is understood or not.

Other than conventional drugs, homeopathic products are the only form of officially regulated medicine in the United States. Homeopathic remedies are usually given as a single dose dissolved under the tongue. Because the remedy stimulates the "vital force" of the body toward healing, the changes are usually gentle and subtle. When the healing forces are stimulated, about 40% of people will notice a temporary increase in some symptoms. This, according to homeopathic knowledge, is a sign of strong healing action.

Some homeopathic remedies may contain alcohol. Of course, you would not want to give your child alcohol. You can, however, heat the mixture and the alcohol will vaporize (boil off). Homeopathic remedies are also made up diluted with water and can be used without heating.

Homeopaths report having good results in treating the fear and anxiety that go along with anticipation of the dental visit. Three medicines are thought to be most commonly effective:

Aconite (monkshood) is given to children for their fear of dentists. It is useful when fear is accompanied by great panic. It is also for those who are restless and angry (and tend to stamp their feet and kick) or are very sensitive to touch.

Gelsemium (yellow jasmine) is given when there is fear along with a feeling of weakness (especially in the stomach), drowsiness, loss of memory, and diarrhea. Gelsemium is also given to children who tend to be hypokinetic (staying too still, with little movement).

Argenicum nitricum (silver nitrate) is given to children who tend to be hyperkinetic (overactive). It is also useful for patients who experience tremor and trembling of the whole body, who tend to be particularly talkative and hurried in their actions, and who have an inner nervousness that affects the bladder and intestines.

For toothaches that result from a dental abscess, some of the common medicines are:

Belladonna (deadly nightshade) is given where there isn't much swelling, but there is much throbbing and redness.

Hepar sulf (Hahnemann's calcium sulfur) is used in the later stages of abscess when pus has formed. The tooth affected is hypersensitive to touch and to cold, and the gums bleed easily.

Silicea (silica) is used after the pus has discharged; it helps healing.

NOTE: Although these medicines may be helpful in alleviating the pain and in some instances in curing, it is often necessary for the abscess to be drained and cared for by the dentist.

For toothaches where there is nerve pain, several medicines are:

Chamomilla is given to those who tend to be very sensitive to warm food and drink, and their symptoms are worse at night. It is good for people overly sensitive to pain.

Coffea is used for those who are so frantic with pain that they cannot sleep, whose pains are also relieved by holding cold water or ice in the mouth, and who are not relieved by *Chamomilla*.

Plantago (plantain) is one of the more common medicines used when there is a toothache with radiating pains to the ears along with facial pain and headache. Homeopaths usually use the tincture or low potencies for the best results from this medicine.

Dr. George Baldwin, an Oakland, California, dentist, Dr. Philip Parsons, a Keystone Heights, Florida, dentist, and Dr. Richard Fischer, an Annandale, Virginia, dentist, have all reported impressive results using *Ruta* (rue) for people who have pain after dental surgery. *Ruta* is known in homeopathy as a great medicine for injuries to the bone and periosteum (the bone covering). *Calendula* (marigolds) is useful in speeding the healing of dental surgery, and is also valuable in healing trauma from injuries to the mouth. It is used for children whose braces irritate their gums or mouth (getting the braces adjusted will also be necessary). Burns from ingesting extremely hot food or drinks are also helped by *Calendula*. If the tincture isn't readily available, making a tea of marigolds is as effective.

Bach Flower Essences

Edward Bach was a medical doctor who didn't like the way that the medical society was treating patients. He read about the work of Hahnemann, the founder of homeopathy. Bach was amazed that Hahnemann had discovered, 100 years before, what he too believed—that doctors should treat the patient, not the disease. Inspired by Hahnemann, Bach went on to develop 38 remedies (called essences) made from wildflowers. The Bach flower remedies were designed to correct emotional imbalances by replacing negative emotions with positive feelings. Dr. Bach discovered that each patient's emotional outlook was different.

The Bach Flower Essences are a safe and natural method of healing. They were designed to gently restore the balance between mind and body and to allow peace and happiness to return to the sufferer so that the body is free to heal itself.

Bach Flower Essences can be used for children. You should read the flower remedy literature (see Bibliography) and the flower remedy self-help questionnaires for additional information on use. The essences are usually prepared using brandy. But you can put the drops into boiling water, which should evaporate the alcohol, making it suitable for children or those who don't like the alcohol content. Flower remedies may be chosen for children of all ages by carefully reading each remedy description and fitting the remedy to the situation. Some remedies that are useful are:

Aspen: helps children deal with unknown fears—something that frightens the child and which he or she cannot identify. It is used for nightmares and hypersensitivity.

Cherry Plum: helps children who have screaming fits and tantrums.

Impatiens: for the child's obvious impatience with delays in having their needs met.

Larch: when the child displays a lack of self-confidence, and does not venture forward.

Mimulus: helps children who are afraid of known things such as going to sleep in the dark, being alone, dogs, and starting school. It is also for shy children.

Rock Rose: for nightmares or when a child becomes terrified or hysterical.

Vervain: helps hyperactive children to be calmer.

Vine: when the child's tantrums seem more like an exercise of power used to get their own way.

Walnut: helps children in periods of change, such as during teething, puberty, new school, new sibling and other situations of change.

Wild Rose: used when the child seems indifferent and apathetic toward circumstances and things.

The Mittlemans kept a bottle of Dr. Bach's Rescue Remedy, a combination of several of the essences, in each of their treatment rooms. All we needed to do was put a few drops on the patient's tongue for fast stress relief. Patients loved the remedy's calming effects.

Other remedies can be chosen by carefully reading and familiarizing yourself with the descriptions of all 38 of the remedies, and using them properly. There are also health professionals who can counsel in the use of the remedies. In all conditions requiring medical attention, a physician or appropriate health care professional should be notified.

Helpful Ways to Reduce Stress

We know that the brain is very powerful. Mental stress can produce chemicals that increase feelings of pain and decrease our natural defenses against it. This is true for children as well as for adults. Coping with discomfort or pain can be more difficult for children, because they cannot express themselves verbally as well as an adult can. All of us—parent, dentist, and the dental staff—have to be alert for opportunities to help a child get through what may be a very distressing situation. We offer some ways to help you help your child have a better dental experience.

The Work of Haim Ginott

Dr. Haim Ginott was a psychologist who wrote many books on parenting and children. His ideas for teachers, as well as parents, apply also in the dentist's office. These ideas can help redirect the rebellious or uncooperative behavior of a child for a better outcome. It can help terrified children to cope with dental treatment. The dentist must use certain words and ideas in conversation with the child. When the child first visits the dentist (and before he or she is put in the dental chair), his or her feelings should be acknowledged. If the child is happy, the dentist should say, "You look happy to be here today; we are happy to see you." More likely, the child will be afraid or uncooperative. The dentist might say, "You look unhappy about being here today. I'll bet you didn't want to come and that you want to go home right now!" A child who sees that you understand how he or she feels may be willing to stop crying and become interested in what the dentist has to say. Then, if the dentist also explains exactly what is to be done, the child will be more trusting and less likely to be uncooperative.

Another way to help the child is to agree with what he or she says—to sympathize. If it's obvious that the child doesn't want to cooperate, the dentist might say, "I wish you didn't have to be here today and were home playing with your friends," or, "I wish I didn't have to count your teeth or take pictures of them." The dentist might also add, "Sometimes grown-ups don't like to go to the dentist." By wishing for the child what he or she wants, we show that we understand. Then, asking for cooperation will usually result in the dentist's getting it.

Children have feelings, but adults don't always consider them. Saying "please" and "thank you" as well as other signs of courtesy should be routine treatment of children. It they are treated like adults, they may act like adults. Children like respect and may not want to lose it by misbehaving. Dr. Ginott also felt that the most important rule is that praise be given for a child's efforts and accomplishments, not for character and personality. For example, if a child is told he is stupid or "bad" at home, what will he think if the dentist tells him that he is smart and "good"? But if the dentist says, "Johnny, you made it easy for me to take care of your teeth today; I want to thank you," then the child is getting praised for what he actually did. It's not a good idea for the parent to say, "You've been such a good boy"; this gives the child the idea that he just went through an ordeal. The next time he might want to act like it really was an ordeal in order to get the same reception.

Dr. Ginott also believed in giving children choices. A dentist using Dr. Ginott's methods would say, "Would you like us to count your top or bottom teeth first?" "Shall we treat the right or left side first?" "Would you like to rest for a minute?" This tells the child that the dentist knows that the child's feelings are important and meaningful. Always look for a way to give the child credit. Most of the world is eager to say "no" to children and point out their faults, says Dr. Ginott. Children need to be liked and need to be told they are liked. Just the dentist's saying, "I like you. You made it easy for me to treat your tooth today," can result in great cooperation next time. If a dentist (or a teacher, or a parent) uses all of the above ideas when dealing with a child, the result is likely to be a big improvement in that child's behavior. Everyone—child, parent, and dentist—will be a lot happier!

Good Nutrition

Dr. Jerome Mittelman and Beverly Mittelman developed methods over the years that can help you and your child be more comfortable during dental visits—without drugs. One of the most important things they found has to do with nutrition. Many people visit the doctor with an empty stomach, probably because blood tests are done. But it's different with the dentist. As we mentioned above, not eating can give you low blood sugar. An insufficient amount of sugar getting to the brain causes irritability, increased sensitivity to pain, and difficulties with handling anesthesia or other medications. This is a good reason *not* to give anesthesia or drugs to children and to try more natural methods. Some smart dentists serve a protein drink to their patients when they arrive for treatment. This is really a kindness. The drink helps normalize sugar levels and raises the body's resistance to stress and infection. Drinks with caffeine taken before or during the visit are not good substitutes for a good breakfast or a protein drink in the dentist's office. Caffeine, whether it's in soda pop, hot chocolate, chocolate milk, tea, or coffee, will first raise blood sugar levels. Very quickly, however, the blood sugar levels will drop even further, resulting in low energy, fatigue, and irritability. This happens because caffeine stimulates the release of insulin from the pancreas. A big burst of insulin will knock blood sugar levels even lower. If the caffeine-containing drink is combined with a carbohydrate food (such as bread, cereal, or doughnuts) the result will be magnified, and extremely low blood sugar will follow. Protein (and fats) will stop this drop in blood sugar levels. Having eggs, cottage cheese, sliced cheese, nuts, meat, or fish before an office visit will prevent low blood sugar and the difficulties that go with it. One patient who learned this lesson asked, "What did *you* have for breakfast today, Dr. Mittelman?"

We talked about sugar in detail in chapter 7 and about a good diet in chapter 8. Sugar, besides being harmful for your child's teeth, can also cause behavior problems in some children. Like caffeine, concentrated sugar such as that in cookies, cakes, sweetened cereals, and beverages can cause low blood sugar by stimulating excess insulin release. In addition to causing low blood sugar, high-sugar foods can also cause hyperactivity in some children. Three to 4 hours after high-sugar meals, some children can become overactive and excited, even emotionally out of control. These spells can last an hour or so. What happens is that in response to the high release of insulin, the body makes epinephrine to counteract the insulin and bring blood sugar levels back up. Epinephrine (also known as adrenaline) is a stimulant. As we mentioned above, local anesthetic injections usually contain epinephrine along with the painkiller. This may compound the problem. For children who are sensitive to high-sugar meals, more complex carbohydrates such as whole-grain cereals, vegetables, and fruit should be included (along with protein) for meals. Complex carbohydrates are not absorbed as quickly into the bloodstream and do not cause such a large increase in insulin as refined sugars.

Many children also have bad responses to food additives such as artificial food coloring, sulfites, and other chemicals mentioned in chapter 8. A meal of natural, wholesome foods will go a long way toward helping your child cope effectively with the dental visit.

A Good Environment

There are some things to do in the dentist's office that can make your child more comfortable. Studies have been done showing that fluorescent lighting has negative effects on our health. The dentist needs fluorescent overhead lighting in order to see well. However, try not to look directly at the light. Ask your child to look to one side or close his or her eyes. The doctor's lamp, the one that shines directly into the mouth, has a positive effect and helps to overcome the negative effects of the overhead lights.

Another good way to help your child relax is to tell him or her to clasp hands on their belly—or maybe on a stuffed animal sitting on it. This is much more calming than gripping the armrests. Also, keeping the legs uncrossed seems to increase calmness. Try not to wear strong perfume or cologne. This may stress the dentist as well as your child.

Anxious mothers (or fathers) can transmit fears to their child. Remember, a positive attitude is contagious—it just might make things easier for your child.

CHAPTER 10

Fluoride: How Safe?
How Effective?

PROMINENT RESEARCHER APOLOGIZES
FOR PUSHING FLUORIDE

Dr. Hardy Limeback, a scientist with impeccable creden-
tials and Canada's leading fluoride authority, upon studying
the lastest research on fluoride, has had a complete reversal of
his formerly favorble position on the use of fluoride. He now
considers it "Poisoning our children . . . ," and as far as stopping cavities, "Here in Toronto, we've been fluoridating for 36
years. Yet Vancouver—which has never fluoridated—has a
cavity rate lower than Toronto's."

Upon being asked why dentists still extol the use of fluoride, Dr. Limeback stated firmly, "Your well-intentioned dentist
is simply following 50 years of misinformation from public
health and the dental association. Me, too. Unfortunately, we
were wrong." (Barry Forbes, *Mesa (Ariz.) Tribune,* Sunday,
December 5, 1999)

Fluoride is a chemical compound at the center of a long-brewing
controversy over its value. At this time, more than 50% of the U.S.
population is drinking fluoridated water from municipal water supplies. This compound is composed of fluorine and another substance such as calcium, tin, or sodium and used for a number of

industrial purposes. Whether it is safe for ingestion by human beings is still not known, despite government claims for its safety. Let's look at some of the facts behind the controversy.

Sodium fluoride (an industrial by-product) is used in toothpaste, dental treatments, and drinking water. If you look in an encyclopedia *(Microsoft Encarta Encyclopedia 2000)* you will find that it is "extremely poisonous." In industry, sodium fluoride is used as an insecticide, particularly for roaches and ants. It is also used to make ceramics, to disinfect equipment in breweries, to preserve wood, and to make paper. Veterinarians use it to deworm animals. Your local government puts it in your water supply, and your dentist puts it in your mouth—supposedly to prevent cavities.

But water fluoridation is still opposed by some people. Reasons for opposition include concerns about possible long-term harmful effects such as a higher risk of osteoporosis (C. Christianson, et al. Effect of fluoride treatment on the fracture rate in postmenopausal women with osteoporosis, *New England Journal of Medicine,* 1990; 332(12): 802–809) And there are objections to "mass medication" without choice. Are there other reasons?

Here's one. Depending on the amount of sodium fluoride used, it can cause anything from ugly teeth to death. Less than 1 gram can cause severe symptoms such as nausea, vomiting, stomach pain, diarrhea, stupor, and weakness. In high amounts (5 to 10 grams) it can cause death. Long-term (chronic) lower-level exposure can cause fluorosis, or mottling of tooth enamel.

The danger to you and to your child is that no one is keeping track of how much fluoride is getting into our bodies from the environment and from what we put into our mouths. The authors of this book believe that you should have all the facts so that you can make the best choice for your child.

According to Ming-Ho Yu, Ph.D., of the Center for Environmental Science at Western Washington University in Bellingham, WA., "The fluoride found in nature isn't readily absorbed by the human body. . . . Sodium fluoride, however, is almost 100% soluble and is absorbed at much greater levels. Children are most at risk, since developing bones absorb more fluoride than those of adults." According to Dr. Yu, fluoride accumulates in the body.

In the 1950s, any toothpaste containing fluoride had to carry a warning label saying that the toothpaste should not be used if local water was fluoridated. This warning disappeared in the late 1950s.

As for giving children supplements of fluoride, researchers say that such supplements should be given only to children at an elevated risk of getting cavities. "Before prescribing them, careful consideration should be given to other fluoride sources, including home and child-care water supplies, foods, and beverages." (W.J.J. Levy, Systemic Fluoride. Sources, amounts, and effects of ingestion *Dental Clinics of North America,* 1999; 43(4) : 695–711).

In very small amounts, fluoride is not toxic—but there is a lot of fluoride in your child's environment. Children also have immature detoxification systems. Their livers cannot handle a dose of fluoride that an adult could detoxify. Try to become aware of the sources of fluoride so your child will never be in danger from an overdose.

On July 2, 1997, the union that consists of and represents all of the biologists, toxicologists, chemists, engineers, and attorneys at the Environmental Protection Agency (EPA) headquarters in Washington, D.C., voted unanimously to take a stand against water fluoridation. They gave scientific evidence of fluoride's link to increased hip fractures, cancers, bone diseases, genetic mutations, and neurological problems, including lower IQ in children. There is also evidence linking fluoride to Alzheimer's disease, kidney damage, chronic fatigue symptoms, and sleep disorders. Other interesting information is that 98% of European countries and Japan do not fluoridate water supplies.

Back before there was fluoride in toothpaste, it was decided that water could contain 1 ppm (part per million) of fluoride and this would give a child who drank a liter of water a day one milligram (mg) of fluoride. No one considered that a small child would have greater effects from one milligram than a larger child has, or that a child could drink more than one liter of water a day. Even at one mg a day, health professionals knew that 10% of all children would have fluoride poisoning.

As far as the Citizens for Safe Drinking Water can determine, no community has gone ahead with fluoridation after officials have completed an accurate study of their own community's total exposure to fluoride. This type of study includes exposure to fluoride from all foods, beverages, air, oral care products, pesticide residues (many of which contain fluoride), and the level of water fluoridation. If a community is already receiving the goal of 1 mg/day from all sources, why would health-conscious professionals still be pushing for fluoridation? One reason is that the National Academy of Sciences (NAS) had classified fluoride as an essential nutrient.

Thanks to a coalition of concerned scientists, important scientific data was entered into the record of the NAS: fluoride's harmful effects, overdosing of fluoride in America, the bone-weakening effects of fluoride, and a report on recent fluoride studies showing no meaningful difference in dental cavities, whether water was fluoridated or nonfluoridated. They pointed out that NAS had made arithmetic and reasoning errors, leading to wrong conclusions about acceptable fluoride levels.

> Fertility rates appear to be lowest in U.S. counties with the highest levels of fluoride, according to a study of nine states.

Are those of us who drink fluoridated water part of a big experiment being conducted without our permission? Physicians, pediatricians, and dentists are not allowed to prescribe ¼, ½, or 1 mg of fluoride drops or tablets without first considering a patient's weight, growth and development, total exposure to fluoride from all sources, and individual susceptibility to fluoride. And yet all of us, our children, and even our infants are getting dosed with fluoride without anyone checking these things—we are being medicated against our will. We should have the right to choose for ourselves what foods we will eat and drink, and what medications we will accept.

Does Research Support the Use of Fluoride?

The truth is that there is no good research to show that putting fluoride in the water supply decreases the rate of tooth decay in children. And it has never even been proven to be safe. Even the discovery that fluoride could affect tooth decay started off on the wrong foot.

Before 1945, scientists were trying to find out why children had stained teeth in Colorado and Texas. They noticed that some of these children with disfigured teeth had fewer cavities than children with normal teeth. They found out that the tooth discoloration was due to naturally high levels of fluoride in the drinking water in these states. On the other hand, there was political incentive to fluoridate the U.S. water supply. Politicians could say, "Look voters, I am helping your children by lobbying for fluoridation."

The Public Health Service never finished the studies that were supposed to show the benefits of fluoride in drinking water. They stopped, because in some of the cities without fluoride, children had **fewer** cavities. They just dropped these cities from their reports—an action that would get any other scientist thrown out of the scientific community or even prosecuted.

Towns and cities could get federal funding to upgrade their water supply systems so that fluoride could be handled. Big business thought it was great to get rid of waste product fluoride cheaply. Yes, the fluoride in our drinking water is a waste product of fertilizer production! No one seemed to care about the facts. Many dentists, doctors, and other health professionals believed what was spoon-fed to them and got on the bandwagon.

If fluoride does any good in preventing tooth decay, it only works on children until about age 13 because it is only incorporated into growing teeth. So why does everyone from 13 on up to 99 have to be exposed to fluoride?

In most European countries, including Finland, Sweden, Denmark, Holland, and France, fluoride is considered a health risk and has been banned. Most of the world has rejected fluoridation. Only America, where it originated, and countries under strong American influence persist in the practice.

Fluoride may be a carcinogen. In 1977, a study was released that linked fluoridation to 10,000 cancer deaths per year in the United

States. The researchers were Dr. John Yiamouyiannis and Dr. Dean Burk, former chief chemist at the National Cancer Institute. Their study showed a 5% increase in cancer rates in cities having fluoridated water supplies.

When all the research finally came in, the result was that rats and mice got rare forms of cancer—osteosarcomas and a rare type of liver cancer, hepatocholangiocarcinoma. The odds of this liver cancer occurring by chance are 1 in 2 million in male mice. Rats and mice also had fluorosis of the teeth, and female rats had osteosclerosis of the long bones. There were also precancerous changes in cells in the mouth and thyroid.

A 1990 *New York Times* article said about the findings, "Previous animal tests suggesting that water fluoridation might pose risks to humans have been widely discounted as technically flawed, but the latest investigation carefully weeded out sources of experimental or statistical error, many scientists say, and cannot be discounted." The *Medical Tribune*, a respected newspaper for physicians, suggested that the Environmental Protection Agency covered up the results. Did the study make any difference in what public health officials told the public? No. The American Dental Association came out with the usual comment that the amount of fluoride used in the animal studies was too high. This is nonsense. The federal government itself, in the *Federal Register* (their book of rules), backs up the practice of giving higher doses to animals when testing for toxicity. Higher doses are given to animals because they don't live as long as humans do, and because humans are usually more vulnerable to toxic substances than animals. If this is the wrong way to do research, then thousands and thousands of experiments done for years by scientists will have to be thrown out! The public, however, was told that everything was fine and not to worry about fluoride. Politics won out over scientific evidence.

Is it just rats that are getting cancer? The New Jersey Department of Health reported in 1992 that osteosarcoma (bone cancer) rates were three to seven times higher in humans in its fluoridated areas than in its nonfluoridated areas. The FDA admitted that they had no studies showing the safety or effectiveness of fluoride.

According to the Holistic Dental Association (see resources), fluoridating any municipal water violates the Safe Drinking Water

Act, the Public Water Systems Act, the Toxic Substances Control Act, and the Drug Cosmetic Act. It's simple: if your local government has approved water fluoridation in your town, they are practicing medicine without a license.

Having Second Thoughts?

Even the people who support fluoridation have some warnings. The American Dental Association does not endorse oral fluoride supplements for infants younger than 6 months of age, regardless of the fluoride level of the drinking water, because an increased incidence of fluorosis has been seen in infants younger than 6 months who received fluoride supplementation. The American Dental Association also states that oral fluoride supplementation should begin at 6 months only if the drinking water supply has fluoride levels less than 0.6 parts per million (ppm) and the infant's caries risk has been determined by health professionals.

The Toothpaste Warning

The American Dental Association says children under 6 should use only a pea-sized amount of fluoride toothpaste on the toothbrush. Unlike what you see in the thousands of TV commercials where toothpaste is spread all over the brush, almost every manufacturer tells parents (on the toothpaste label) to use the pea-sized amount and to supervise young children to make sure the tiny drop used in brushing is completely spit out.

The Food and Drug Administration (FDA) requires toothpaste companies to add a warning telling parents to seek professional advice or contact a poison control center if a child swallows too much toothpaste. The FDA admits that adverse reactions such as fluorosis or overdose can occur. For all fluoride gels, pastes and powders they say: "WARNING: Keep out of reach of children under 6 years of age. In case of accidental overdose, seek professional assistance or contact a poison control center immediately."

Why would you want to put something so dangerous in your child's mouth? Can you be 100% sure that your child will never swallow a gob of toothpaste? What about the whole tube? Are you going to lock up the toothpaste? Even an amount covering the bristles of a toothbrush contains 1 milligram of fluoride, which is four times the daily dose recommended for children up to age 3.

But how much is too much? The Centers for Disease Control (CDC) found that children are exposed to fluoride from many sources, including drinking water, toothpaste, fluoride supplements, and even grape juice. "There probably is excess exposure," says Kit Shaddix, fluoride team leader with the CDC's division of oral health. This may be due to the fact that some well-meaning parents often put a large glob of toothpaste on their children's toothbrush. The message of the pea-sized amount has not gotten across, according to Dr. Shaddix, who blames the toothpaste ads showing generous amounts of toothpaste squeezed onto the brush. He also says that pediatricians and dentists routinely give children fluoride supplements in areas where the water is fluoridated. "Put those two together, and you could get a big problem with fluorosis," says Dr. Shaddix.

There were 12,000 calls to the poison control centers in 1997 over swallowed fluoride, mostly for children acutely poisoned by too much toothpaste or mouthwash. Chronic low-dose exposure, however, is a very serious problem which has not been addressed at this time. Does fluoride toothpaste alone, when used in the early years of life, cause fluorosis? It's hard to tell in developed countries where a child may be exposed to many sources of fluoride.

One way to tell is to look at children whose only potential source of fluoride was fluoride toothpaste. A study was done on 1,189 children in Goa, India, whose only source of fluoride was the toothpaste they used. The researchers found that among children with fluorosis, beginning brushing with fluoride toothpaste before the age of 2 years increased the severity of fluorosis significantly.

Some children like the taste of toothpaste so much that they eat it. Research indicates that many young children swallow 100% of the toothpaste on their brush. Some disabled children cannot completely spit out all of the toothpaste. Parents of children who use fluoridated toothpaste might want to keep the telephone number of the poison control center nearby until the child learns how to spit the toothpaste out!

Some toothbrush manufacturers are trying to help parents by

making the head of the toothbrush smaller and putting colored bristles to show them where to put the toothpaste.

Fluoride in Water and Other Beverages

Starting with baby foods, there is more fluoride than you would think in many foods and beverages. An article published in the *Journal of the American Dental Association* told how high levels of fluoride in some infant foods could put babies at risk for dental fluorosis. The researchers analyzed the fluoride concentration of 206 ready-to-eat infant foods and 32 dry infant cereals, prepared with water (nonfluoridated) according to the manufacturer's directions. They found that cereals, fruits, and vegetables had the lowest levels of fluoride, while foods with chicken had the highest fluoride levels.

In very small amounts, fluoride can be used in the body. A baby drinking only breast milk gets some fluoride. This small amount, according to the La Leche League, ". . . seems to be perfectly suited to the baby's need."

Fluoridated water added to dry baby foods also increases the levels of fluoride babies are getting. "Any infants who regularly eat more than a couple of ounces of infant foods containing high-fluoride-content chicken would be at elevated fluorosis risk," write the researchers. Babies eating these foods should not be getting fluoride from other sources such as toothpaste, supplements, or water.

The chicken has high fluoride (about 1 ppm) because bits of chicken skin and bone, which contain fluoride, get into the baby food during mechanical processing. The researchers also found out that different types of baby foods had a variety of amounts of fluoride. The level depended on what water source was used in preparing the food at the factory.

In a study where juices and juice blends were tested, it was found that 42% of the samples had more than 1 ppm of fluoride, with some brands of grape juice containing up to 6.8 ppm. These high levels come from the use of fluoride-containing insecticides used in growing grapes. There are no warning labels on these juices that contain more than the 1 ppm "acceptable" amount of fluoride.

"It's important for parents to know how much fluoride their children are getting, whether it's through the water supply, fluoride supplements, fluoridated toothpaste or baby food," said the researchers. One of the researchers, Dr. Gary M. Whitford, said that fluoride could be toxic in very large doses. If a small child doubled up on the amount of toothpaste that the toothbrush normally holds, and swallowed, it might cause a stomach upset, according to Whitford. However, if a child ate a whole tube, Whitford would call poison control, or better still, the hospital because, he says, poisoning develops very quickly. "There's one case we had where the child died in 3 hours, and there are other cases where they died a few days later, depending on the dose," said Whitford.

Dr. Michael Easley, spokesperson for the American Dental Association and associate professor in the School of Dental Medicine at the State University of New York at Buffalo, says, "Parents really need to sit down with their dentist or pediatrician and try to decide how much fluoride the infant might be getting based on the amount of those kinds of foods the baby is eating. . . . If fluoride content is not on the label, it should be."

Most people think that the fluoride content of bottled water is insignificant. Studies show, however, that varying amounts are present, and some are rather high. Some juices and infant formulas and foods have also been reported to have high levels of fluoride.

Doctors and dentists must consider that beverages such as grape juice and tea may contain more fluoride than fluoridated water. Colas, soft drinks, and juices bottled in areas where water is fluoridated also contain fluoride. It hasn't happened yet, but the FDA is calling for labeling rules listing the fluoride content of the food or beverage.

Cooking food in fluoridated water of course raises the fluoride content of the food. So it is important to consider all the sources of fluoride in a child's environment.

One other source of fluoride is dental sealants. Although sealants can be beneficial to your child, some contain fluoride, such as Helioseal F. The "F" stands for . . . what else but fluoride! Only the manufacturer of the sealant, and perhaps the Food and Drug Administration, knows how much F is in the sealant. Ask the manufacturer. Surely they were required to answer these questions before they were allowed to sell a time-release poisonous drug such as fluoride to innocent people.

Fluorosis

The American Academy of Pediatric Dentistry will tell you that too much fluoride during tooth development will cause fluorosis. The fluoride causes defects in the tooth enamel; in mild cases, there are white specks or streaks. In severe cases, new teeth can come up chalky white. In both cases, the teeth are weak and parts of the enamel may break away. Later, the teeth will have discoloration or brown markings.

Once fluoride is part of the tooth enamel, it can't be taken out. There are some cosmetic dental treatments for teeth, but teeth aren't the only things affected. Fluoride gets into bones and soft tissues all over the body. It can cause muscle wasting, spine deformities, brain disturbances and calcium deposits in ligaments. If it hasn't been reported much, this is because most doctors aren't taught about the disease and don't know how to recognize it when they see it. Even more frightening are reports from China that children with fluorosis have lower intelligence scores. In the United States, animal studies showed that fluoride accumulates in the brain and affects behavior and the ability to learn.

Dr. Dean Edell, the physician seen on TV and also on the web site HealthCentral, talked about fluoride: "Too much fluoride can harm the teeth, especially in young children. The result—fluorosis of the teeth . . . and this ugly discoloration can be permanent." Dr. Edell says that dentists are seeing an increase in cases of dental damage from excess fluoride.

According to a report of the U.S. Preventive Service Task Force, fluorosis has been increasing. However, the report states that this is because of the inappropriate use of fluoride supplements by health professionals and parents—not from fluoride in the water supply.

The Task Force does not recommend fluoride for children under 3 years of age, even in areas where there is little or no fluoride in the water supply.

A Mother's Sad Story

Darlene Sherrell had a sad story to tell. She told it on the Internet so that people could learn from her and perhaps prevent their children from a similar fate. Her daughter Julie couldn't be nursed because of problems Darlene had with nursing. Julie couldn't drink formula without getting sick. The only thing she could keep down was a powdered formula that Darlene mixed with fluoridated water. Of course Darlene was not aware of the dangers of too much fluoride. Julie's baby teeth crumbled within 30 minutes of emerging from her gums, according to Darlene.

In the third grade Julie has a spontaneous fracture of her ankle and her X-rays had a Swiss cheese appearance. Darlene was told that it was common and didn't mean anything. Julie's thyroid then became enlarged and returned to normal several times around puberty. By the age of 17 she had developed thyroid cancer. Finally, in 1976 Darlene heard about the dangers of fluoride. When Darlene saw X-rays of children with fluorosis she realized how similar they were to her daughter's X-rays. No one wanted to help her. No laboratory in the country would analyze the fallen-out baby teeth that Darlene had saved—they didn't want to get involved. Also, no city, county, state, or national agency would accept a report of fluoride poisoning. So Darlene started her own newsletter and organized classes to teach people about organic gardening and health. She spent several months reading the research papers used by the health department to figure out the amount of fluoride that would cause fluorosis. She found that when the fluoride amount was calculated, a math mistake was made. With this information she convinced state legislators and the Michigan Department of Public Health that there was a problem. She helped bring about a repeal of the state mandatory fluoridation law.

A Dental Assistant Speaks Out

Patti Gibbons works as a dental assistant in Woodcliff Lake, New Jersey. She researched and wrote about fluoride while still in school. According to Patti, she wanted information that would "help us judge whether we feel confident having it used as a treatment in preventing tooth decay." She came across a study where people living in Arizona, Colorado, Illinois, Iowa, New Mexico, Ohio, South Dakota, and Texas had mottled teeth, or dental fluorosis.

The damage to their teeth ranged from a mild case of having small white specks on the enamel, to more severe cases where the enamel was discolored and pitted, exposing the underlayer of dentin. The problem was traced to the water supply, which had a high concentration of naturally occurring fluoride. She found information that fluoride toothpaste can be dangerous to your child's health. Children between the ages of 2 and 6 tend to swallow 35% of their toothpaste when a normal amount is applied to their toothbrush. Not only can this amount cause nausea and a stomach ache, but a child could be swallowing up to 1 milligram or more of fluoride at each brushing.

She found a report that stated, "Fluoride is considered more toxic than lead and is fatal in high doses. A single dose of five grams is lethal to an adult and one gram or less, to a small child, and as little as four to eight milligrams taken into the body daily, while enamel is forming, can cause dental fluorosis." (One thousand milligrams equals one gram.)

Unfortunately, unlike adults, children cannot eliminate excess fluoride through feces or urine. Many foods contain fluoride.

FLUORIDE CONTENT OF SOME FOODS (MICROGRAMS IN 100 GRAMS OF EDIBLE PORTION)

Almonds	90	Eggs, whole	118
Apples	5–132	Frankfurters	167
Banana	23	Grape juice	9
Beef	29–200	Milk	10–55

Butter	150	Oranges	7–17
Carrots	40	Rice	10–67
Cheese	162	Spinach	20–180
Chicken	140	Strawberry	18
Codfish	700	Tuna	10

Patti Gibbons concluded: "The facts are clear about fluoride. It has proven itself to be extremely controversial and it is here to stay indefinitely. But we can control certain amounts ingested through our diets by educating ourselves as to what foods contain fluoride, learning about how much fluoride is in our water, our drugs, and vitamins. It is important to have good communication with the dentist, pediatrician, family doctor, and pharmacist in determining how much fluoride is too little or too much. It is good to be skeptical."

How Much Is Too Much?

How much is too much fluoride? The probable toxic dose is about 5 milligrams of fluoride for each 2.2 pounds of body weight. For a 2-year-old child weighing about 25 pounds, this would be 57 grams. Two ounces of a 1,000 ppm toothpaste, 8 ounces of a 0.5% sodium fluoride mouth rinse, and less than a teaspoon of 1.23% acidulated phosphate fluoride gel contain this toxic amount. How many children have eaten 2 ounces of toothpaste?

Fluoride toothpaste can contain 1,000–1,500 ppm, which can cause gum damage, sickness—or even death if a small child eats a family-sized tube. Even fluoride mouth rinse sold in stores or given in schools can contain 500 ppm fluoride, enough to cause sickness.

In Brooklyn, New York, in January 1979, a three-year-old boy died from fluoride overdose. It happened when the dental hygienist was cleaning his teeth. She swabbed his teeth with a fluoride gel that is supposed to be left on briefly and rinsed out. She gave the boy a cup of water and never told him to wash his mouth out and spit out the gel. The child drank the water and swallowed all of the gel. His stomach was not pumped out in time, and he went into a coma and died.

Fluoride treatments done by the dentist can contain 5,000 to 20,000 ppm fluoride. When a young child gets a fluoride treatment in the dentist's office the child is expected to hold a highly toxic dose of fluoride in his or her mouth for 5 minutes. Can every child do this without swallowing any of the fluoride? How many parents are told that if their child swallows the fluoride gel the child could die? These are questions that need answers before you expose your child to fluoride. We have given you the facts on fluoride and answered many questions about its use. Now it's up to you to make the decision.

CHAPTER 11

The Mercury/Silver Filling Controversy

Mercury: A Toxic Metal

Silver fillings may look like silver, but don't judge this book by its cover. "Silver" fillings are really amalgams—mixtures of metals. The most common combination for dental fillings is 52% mercury, 30% copper, 13% tin, 4% silver, and less than 1% zinc. Mercury, the main ingredient, is one of the most poisonous metals known.

Mercury was commonly used years ago as an antiseptic. Before antibiotics, mercury was used to treat syphilis. It was extremely toxic and killed patients—in some cases before the disease did. Some of us will remember "mercurochrome," found in every medicine cabinet and swabbed onto every cut and scrape. The germs in the cut were definitely less of a menace than the mercury absorbed through the skin. If you thought that you could no longer find it on the pharmacy shelf today, think again. It is still there but hiding behind other names.

Thimerosal is a mercury-containing antibacterial chemical that you will find in many, many products. It has been used since the 1930s to kill bacteria and fungi. Thimerosal is known widely as a first-aid product available as "tincture of Merthiolate®" for home use (see Appendixes for other names it goes by). It is used as a preservative in cosmetics, including makeup removers, eye moisturizers, and mascara. It may be found in soap-free cleansers; in nose-, eye-, and eardrops; and in eye ointments, topical medications, and antiseptic sprays. Exposure may occur through the use of cleaning fluids for contact lenses that contain this toxic chemical.

Thimerosal also is used widely as a preservative in vaccines, antitoxins, tuberculin tests, and desensitization solutions. Yes, influenza (flu) vaccine, hepatitis B, and some of the diphtheria and tetanus toxoids and acellular pertussis (DTaP) vaccine given to infants contain thimerosal. In July 1999, the Public Health Service, the American Academy of Pediatrics, and vaccine manufacturers agreed that the use of thimerosal as a preservative should be removed as soon as possible. But they said that vaccines containing thimerosal should still be given to infants, children, and adults because the risk of having the disease was worse than exposure to mercury. Companies that make vaccines are working on taking the thimerosal out. Merck & Co. released a thimerosal-free hepatitis B vaccine on August 27, 1999, and as of this writing other companies were working to take the toxin out of their vaccines. What about all the other products that contain mercury preservatives? Who knows? We haven't seen any companies making efforts to take it out.

We have an immune system to handle germs, but no such effective way to get rid of toxic metals. How many of us played with the liquid mercury from a broken thermometer? Most metals are solids. Mercury is an unusual metal in that it is liquid at room temperature. It is highly volatile, meaning that it turns easily into fumes that can readily be absorbed into the tissues in the nose and lungs. Children especially, with their immature livers and kidneys (the organs that do detoxification in the body), cannot deal with toxic substances. For the unborn, in the development stages of organs, there is practically no protection, not even from the baby's mother. Mercury crosses the placenta. In the form of mercury vapor, the same kind released by mercury amalgam fillings, about 50% of the mercury is taken up by the placenta, passes through it, and enters the fetus. Once in the bloodstream, mercury can get into most tissues in both mother and baby easily. Alcohol will cause increased uptake of mercury vapor by the mother's thyroid and the fetal thyroid and liver.

A study of 418 female dental assistants who prepare 30 or more amalgam fillings per week showed that their fertility was only 63% that of woman not exposed to mercury at work. The effect of mercury amalgam exposure on brain function of dental personnel shows up as problems with attention and perception.

In the 1800s, mercury amalgam was introduced to the United States from England and France. Some dentists became concerned that mercury amalgam was poisonous. By 1845, the American Society of Dental Surgeons and several other affiliated dental organizations had members sign a pledge not to use amalgam. But dentists who wanted to use amalgam won and the society was disbanded in 1856. In its place arose in 1859 the American Dental Association (ADA), who said mercury amalgam was just fine for use as a filling material. For over 150 years we have been told that mercury from fillings can not harm our children, our unborn fetuses, or us. Is this the truth? Let's look at all the facts before we make a decision.

The Dangers of Mercury in Dental Fillings

Jerome Mittelman, D.D.S., stopped using amalgam fillings in 1968. He knew that amalgams had been used for 150 years, but he was convinced the field of dentistry was wrong. When interviewed on ABC, Dr. Mittelman reminded viewers that asbestos was also used for 150 years before its toxicity was realized.

Ask your dentist to sign the following: "I certify that if I place silver amalgam fillings (which contain 50% mercury) in your teeth they will not be harmful to your health."

Leaching Out and Toxic Vapors

People are led to believe—and even most dentists believe—that mixing silver alloy and mercury makes a stable filling that won't release mercury. It's true that when two metals combine *chemically,* the resulting compound is stable. An example would be mixing milk and eggs together and making custard. The milk and eggs won't go back to being milk and eggs. But that's not what happens in amalgam. The mercury is joined *physically* instead. This is like mixing salt and pepper together. It looks like one substance but, if you were patient, you could separate the salt from the pepper. And that's how mercury is mixed with silver and the other metals in the amalgam. It's not stable. It can vaporize at ordinary temperatures. The mercury vapor is released from new fillings as well as from those that have hardened and aged.

It wasn't until the early 1980s that several laboratories showed that mercury vapor is continuously released from amalgam tooth fillings. The researchers found that the rate of release is increased immediately after chewing (7 to 9 micrograms) and tooth brushing (10 micrograms). Continuous chewing for 10 to 30 minutes can raise the oral mercury level as high as 100 micrograms or more. Personal habits such as chewing gum, grinding teeth, and mouth breathing can greatly increase a person's daily exposure to amalgam mercury vapor. Eventually these levels go back down to what they were before chewing and brushing about 90 minutes after stopping. We have more mercury to worry about. According to the World Health Organization, the general sources of mercury in the body are breathed air (.040 micrograms), fish (2.34 micrograms), nonfish food (.25 micrograms), and drinking water (.0035 micrograms). The mercury vapor from dental amalgams alone (3 to 17 micrograms) is still the highest amount.

> In the opinions of mercury toxicity experts Thomas Clarkson of the University of Rochester Medical School in New York and Lars Friberg of the Karolinska Institute in Stockholm, Sweden, there is no safe level of mercury exposure.

Years ago, dentists and the American Dental Association (ADA) assured us that mercury would never leach out of fillings. When more evidence showed that it did leach out, the ADA (in 1981) changed its tune and publicly admitted that mercury leaches from dental fillings. They also told dentists and dental assistants: "Handling amalgams requires extreme caution. . . . a 'no-touch' technique should be employed." We would like to know how they could keep the patient's mouth from touching it! After these announcements, they began saying that patients should not worry—that the amount that leaches out could not hurt anyone. It seems that while the ADA is worried about dentists' exposure to mercury, they are not too concerned about patients' exposure. In the *ADA News* (September 7, 1981) report by the Council on Dental Materials, Instruments, and Equipment was the statement, "Dentists should alert all personnel who handle mercury about the potential hazards of mercury vapor and the need for good mercury hygiene practices." The report listed the symptoms of mercury poisoning (a partial list):

Shaky movements of muscles, such as those used for handwriting
Loss of appetite
Nausea and diarrhea
Depression, fatigue, increased irritability, and moodiness
Insomnia
Swollen glands and tongue
Ulcers in the mouth lining
Birth defects in children of mothers exposed to mercury

The ADA continued: "All amalgam scrap [excess material from silver fillings] should be salvaged and stored in a tightly closed container." They want to keep the vapors from getting to dental personnel. But what about dental patients? The Environmental Protection Agency (EPA) has warned dentists not to release scrap mercury material into sewers. If it's not safe for sewers, why would you want it in your child's mouth?

The ADA also says, "The strongest and most convincing support we have for the safety of dental amalgam is the fact that each year more than 100 million amalgam fillings are placed [in people's teeth] in the United States." What a scary thought! Tons of mercury are being put in people's mouths without any proof of safety! Remember that the symptoms from mercury toxicity are medical symptoms that might be recognized by a doctor, but not by a dentist. People got their mercury fillings, went home, and if they had symptoms, went to their doctors, not back to the dentist. So nobody was making a connection between mercury in fillings and symptoms of toxicity. Because the symptoms mentioned in the list could have other causes, even most doctors would not realize that the cause was the mercury.

On a CBS News *60 Minutes* show on December 16, 1990, Morley Safer reported: "Last summer, the EPA banned mercury from indoor latex paint because of mercury vapor. The vapor level in this patient's mouth after chewing for 10 minutes is 92 times higher than that in a newly painted room, three times higher than the U.S. government allows in the workplace." Safer went on to say that mercury amalgams were never tested for safety because it was assumed that mercury was made stable when mixed with other metals. The Food and Drug Administration automatically approved amalgams based on an assumption—not on real science. Said Safer, "But now a growing number of scientists, doctors, and dentists are saying silver amalgams should be banned. . . . No specific disease has yet been directly linked to mercury from fillings, but now a number of medical schools are looking at the relationship between mercury vapor in the mouth and a whole variety of diseases. Alzheimer's, arthritis, and colitis have all been linked to mercury poisoning. Mercury in the workplace has produced kidney damage, brain damage, birth defects, and symptoms of multiple sclerosis."

On the show, Dr. Murray Vimy, a dentist and a consultant from the World Health Organization, said: "There is no safe threshold for mercury exposure. None. And there isn't someone somewhere who may not have a very violent reaction even to the lowest amounts of mercury." Although Dr. Heber Simmons of the American Dental Association went on to say that the mercury vapor from fillings was at such a low level that it couldn't cause any problems, Dr. Vimy didn't agree. He said that the entire human population in the Western world who has had amalgams is an experiment on the effects of chronic, low-dose exposure to a heavy (toxic) metal and that no one has ever really looked at mercury exposure on such a level. Much is known about exposure to large amounts of mercury in a short time period, but not levels that people get day after day, he explained.

Magnus Nylander, D.D.S., of the Karolinska Institute, Stockholm, Sweden, "presented his findings concerning mercury levels in the brains of dentists at the University of Colorado at Colorado Springs Toxic Element Research Foundation Conference. He reported that autopsies of dentists showed an increase of 800 times over the control level [persons not exposed to mercury] of mercury in the pituitary gland [of the brain].

U.S. Government Document Admits That Mercury Vapors from Silver Fillings Exceed the Minimum Risk Levels Established by the US Department of Health and Human Services!

The facts are now clear. Buried in the 351-page document *Toxicological Profile for Mercury (Update)* May 1994 published by the U.S. Department of Health and Human Services, the scientific truth has finally been divulged. On page 125 of this document it states: "A report from the Committee to Coordinate Environmental Health and Related Programs (CCEHRP) of the Department of Health and Human Services determined that 'measurement of mercury in blood among subjects with and without amalgam restorations . . . and subjects before and after amalgams were removed . . . provided the best estimates of daily intake from amalgam dental restorations. These values are in the range of 1–5 mcg/day (Dept. of Human Health & Services 1993, page III-29). The chronic inhalation Minimal Risk Level is 0.014 mcg/m3. . . . The proposed acute Minimal Risk Level is 0.02 mcg/m_3. Thus, both MRL's are below estimated levels from dental amalgams.' "

Metals are very chemically reactive. When they are mixed together, they can be even more reactive. In the book *Mercury Poisoning from Dental Amalgam: A Hazard to the Human Brain* by Patrick Stortebecker, M.D., Ph.D., is research by A. Gura Knappwost et al. (p. 132), which states that when mixed metals are present in the mouth, like gold crowns and amalgam fillings, a release of mercury occurs that is 10 times higher when compared to amalgam fillings alone.

Mercury Helps Bacteria Thrive

Today, in this country and all over the world, we are faced with the frightening possibility that bacteria will one day be resistant to all the antibiotics currently used to treat infections. It's happening already: as many as half of all bacteria that cause urinary tract infections are now resistant to penicillin and other common antibiotics. Every time an antibiotic is used against bacteria, most of the bacteria are killed—but just a few survive. The bacteria that survive have changes in their genetic material that make them resistant to the antibiotic. Microbiologists have found that mercury in dental fillings helps the bacteria become even more resistant to antibiotics. This happens because the genes that protect bacteria against mercury poisoning are close to the genes that make bacteria resistant to antibiotics. When the bacteria are exposed to mercury, the genes are turned on that help the bacteria change the toxic form of mercury (ionic mercury) into mercury vapor—a less toxic form (for them). In doing this, the nearby genes for antibiotic resistance are also turned on. Even when no antibiotics were given, test animals were found to have increased levels of antibiotic-resistant bacteria in their intestines after having amalgam fillings put in their mouths. Dr. George Jacoby of Harvard Medical School, an expert on antibiotic-resistant bacteria, said that he believes that dental fillings are contributing to the increase in resistant bacteria.

Bacteria in your mouth can convert metallic mercury into another form called methyl mercury. This has been well known since the 1950s. Most strains of staphylococci and streptococci, yeasts, and the bacterium *Escherichia coli* (present in human intestines) are able to do this conversion. Methyl mercury is said to be 100 times more poisonous than elemental mercury. In this form it easily crosses the blood-brain barrier and gets into the brain. The blood-brain barrier is like a gate—it lets some toxic substances and drugs into the brain, but keeps others out. Unfortunately, methyl mercury is one toxic substance that does get in.

What Mercury Can Do to Your Child

Your child's environment is full of toxic substances. Some pollution, like that found in the air and water, you can't do much about. But you can protect your child from mercury toxicity. Say "no" to mercury amalgams! The damage mercury can do to your child can't be repaired.

For any toxic substance, it's common sense to know that the younger and smaller the human being, the worse will be the effects of the poison. So, of course, it is the developing fetus that gets the most severe damage. Since research can't be done on live human fetuses, an experiment was done on sheep to find out just what mercury does to the unborn. The pregnant sheep got 12 mercury amalgam fillings. The mercury was made radioactive so that it could be traced wherever it went in the sheep's bodies and in the bodies of the unborn sheep. After 3 days, mercury was found in the mother sheep's blood, in the amniotic fluid surrounding the fetuses, in fetal blood, and in the mothers' feces and urine. When the researchers checked after 16 days, the mothers' mercury levels were highest in the kidney, liver, gastrointestinal tract, and thyroid. The mercury levels in the fetuses were highest in the pituitary gland of the brain, the liver, kidney and in the placenta. By 33 days, there were higher levels of mercury in the fetuses than in the mothers. The mercury in the fetuses was in the liver, bones, bile, bone marrow, blood, and brain. The mothers could get rid of some of the mercury, but the unborn sheep could not. When the mother sheep were nursing the newborn sheep, there was eight times more mercury in the milk than in the mother's blood. This increased the mercury exposure to the newborn sheep.

The researchers believe the animal research may be a warning about the effects of amalgam in humans. "We know that there's no obvious mortality (death) associated with amalgam," said one of the researchers. "Indeed, there may not be any. But we do know that mercury is highly toxic and that it concentrates in certain parts of the human body. From the sheep, we know it can alter kidney function in animals. That should be enough to get it banned." The researchers also said that these results did not fit with the opinions of the dental profession about the dangers of mercury from fillings. Notice that we said "opinions" of the dental profession. Because that's what they are. There are no good studies, or any studies for that matter, that prove mercury, in any amount, is safe for anyone! The ADA, in its "Statement of Confidence in Amalgam," no longer says that the safety of these fillings has been scientifically proven. All it can say is that mercury has 150 years of "successful" use. So did asbestos—and lead and DDT were also used for years.

On May 20, 1987, the story hit the newspapers in Sweden that the Swedish government had declared that mercury amalgam was toxic and unsuitable as a dental filling material. The first step taken was to eliminate the use of amalgam work on pregnant women in order to prevent mercury damage to the fetus. They said, "We realize now that we have previously made an error in our judgment on this question. Patients have suffered unnecessarily and we will now rectify our mistakes and in different ways try to solve the problem."

One of the properties of mercury that makes it so toxic is that it can easily dissolve in fats. These fats (called lipids) surround all the cells in our bodies. Lipid membranes surround brain cells. So mercury can easily get into your child's brain. Studies that looked at levels of mercury in the brains of fetuses and newborn babies found that the levels were higher the more fillings the mothers had. The part of the brain where mercury accumulated was the cerebral cortex, the area where higher thinking, such as memory, takes place. Mercury also produces brain lesions that resemble the damage seen in Alzheimer's disease.

Mercury, after it leaches from dental fillings, can travel all over the body through the blood. It doesn't do any good to test blood for the level of mercury because the mercury is immediately pulled out of the blood into body tissues. Besides reaching the brain, it can directly affect the immune system. According to Hal Huggins, D.D.S., M.S., a specialist in the removal of mercury fillings and other toxic dental materials, the immune system sees mercury as a challenge. "With the first sign of mercury in the body, the immune system dispatches specialized immune cells, such as leukocytes (white blood cells), lymphocytes, eosinophils, and basophils, to deal with the poison," says Huggins. Keeping the white blood cell count continually high to fight the mercury puts stress on the immune system and it becomes fatigued. A tired immune system cannot do its job. It may not be able to fight germs or cancer cells if it's busy dealing with mercury. It was found that even the silver in the amalgam, by itself, could cause immune stress.

There is some evidence that mercury can cause multiple sclerosis (MS) or make it worse. MS is disease of the brain and spinal cord where nerves become damaged causing muscle weakness, visual loss, paralysis, and mood alterations. There is presently no conventional cure for MS and these persons will eventually die of the disease. (There are, however, holistic doctors who have had success in controlling and even say they can reverse the disease.) One study looked at the blood of people with MS with mercury-containing fillings and those who had their fillings removed. MS subjects with mercury fillings had significantly lower levels of red blood cells and immune system cells, compared to MS patients who had their fillings removed. A health questionnaire found that MS patients with mercury fillings had significantly more (33.7%) flare-ups of MS during a 12-month period compared to the MS volunteers with filling removal. Another study found that patients with multiple sclerosis and mercury fillings had significantly more depression, anger, and other psychiatric problems. According to the authors of the study, the poorer mental health status shown by multiple sclerosis patients with fillings may be associated with mercury toxicity from the amalgam.

Nutrients That Protect Against Mercury

Not ever allowing mercury fillings to be placed in your child's teeth is, of course, the best way to avoid mercury toxicity. However, your child may have already received such a filling or you, as a potential, pregnant, or nursing mother, may have mercury fillings. What can you do? Removing such fillings, even one at a time, can be very dangerous unless done by a dentist trained in the safe removal of toxic mercury. Most certainly, even this should not be done by any woman trying to get pregnant (or her partner) or one who is already pregnant. As we said before, the fetus is most susceptible to the damage from mercury toxicity. Mercury is a "heavy metal" along with lead, cadmium, arsenic, nickel, and aluminum. These types of metals tend to accumulate in the brain, kidneys, and immune system, causing severe disruptions in normal function. We get these heavy metals from industrial pollution, pesticide sprays, cooking utensils, cigarette smoke, antacids, and, for mercury, from dental fillings, contaminated fish, and some cosmetics. With such a burden of heavy metals assaulting our bodies, why would we want to add another by getting mercury fillings?

If we can detoxify mercury and other harmful substances we can make a big difference in how healthy our children and we can be. There are ways to help the body eliminate mercury more quickly or defend against its toxicities by using certain important nutrients. A good nutrient base should be a diet that has lots of fresh fruits (especially oranges and tangerines) and vegetables (especially cabbage, broccoli, Brussels sprouts, peppers, tomatoes, avocados, and asparagus), whole grains, legumes (beans and peas), nuts (including walnuts), and seeds. Such a diet will contain many detoxifying nutrients, including those listed below.

Vitamin C

Vitamin C can have a protective effect against mercury poisoning. Our bodies use it to make one of the most important detoxifying enzymes—glutathione. Glutathione is not very effective when taken by mouth as a supplement (it's not absorbed well), but vitamin C can increase its levels in the body. Foods that are rich in glutathione are those mentioned above: asparagus, avocado, walnuts, cabbage, broccoli, Brussels sprouts, oranges, tangerines, dill, and caraway seeds.

Vitamin C is also a "metal chelator" which means that it wraps around toxic metals, such as mercury and lead, and can pull them out of the body. When guinea pigs were given a lethal dose of mercury, 40% of those that had been given high levels of vitamin C before receiving the mercury survived. In the 1940s, mercury was an ingredient in diuretics (water pills) used by doctors to lower blood pressure. These doctors knew that the toxicity of these mercury diuretics could be reduced if they gave the patient vitamin C before or with the drug. Mercury can also stop collagen synthesis. Collagen is the connective tissue that holds teeth in their sockets and keeps blood vessel walls flexible and healthy. Vitamin C is needed to make collagen. The swollen and bleeding gums seen in vitamin C deficiency (scurvy) are due to poorly made collagen. If there is not enough vitamin C in the diet and the vitamin is being used up to

detoxify mercury from fillings, then gum disease will be the outcome.

Our adrenal glands contain high levels of stored vitamin C. When
we are under stress (mental or physical), we make adrenaline, a
hormone that prepares us for "fight or flight." Adrenaline prepares
us to face the mental or physical challenge. As we make adrenaline,
vitamin C levels fall since the vitamin is used to make the adrenaline. Long-term exposure to low mercury levels depresses the
adrenal vitamin C content. According to Dr. Michael F. Ziff, an expert on mercury toxicity, "The person with amalgam dental fillings
who is being exposed to chronic intakes of mercury vapor would
also be subjecting the adrenals to depletion by chemical stress."

Cysteine, Methionine, and Taurine

Mercury is known to bind to amino acids such as cysteine, methionine, and taurine in the body. These amino acids contain sulfur,
an element that is used in many of the body's detoxifying systems.
Cysteine and methionine are very important in helping our bodies
to detoxify harmful chemicals and drugs. These amino acids are
found in foods such as garlic, onions, and eggs. Sulfur-containing
foods include red peppers, egg yolks, broccoli, and Brussels sprouts.
When mice were given cysteine at the same time as mercury, the
amount of mercury in the animals' bodies (liver and kidneys) was
reduced. Levels of mercury in the brain were not reduced. Before
birth the enzymes necessary to get cysteine into the brain are not
present. So the unborn baby depends on the mother's blood as a
source of cysteine. Taurine is made from cysteine, so it's important
that the mother have a good supply. This sulfur-containing amino
acid is highly concentrated in the brain, where it can protect brain
cells and help them function properly. Taurine also protects the
heart and helps it work better. The amounts of taurine are high in
the fetal liver and brain and some researchers think that taurine
helps brain development.

Zinc

Zinc is a mineral that is very important for growth and development, skin health, and wound repair. It is found in every body cell

and is necessary for proper action of body hormones including those that control growth and sugar levels. It is also needed to make metallothionein, a very important compound that helps us detoxify toxic metals such as mercury, cadmium, and copper. Zinc also supports the function of a healthy immune system. It is found in high amounts in white blood cells that defend the body from germs. High concentrations of zinc are also found in the bone, skin, kidney, liver, pancreas, the retina of the eye, and the prostate. It is essential for male reproductive success. Even with mild zinc deficiency, there is increased susceptibility to infection, poor wound healing, decreased sense of taste or smell, and many skin disorders. Also found are a decreased ability to see at night, slowing of growth, mouth ulcers, a white coating on the tongue, bad breath, and white spots on the fingernails. Zinc is absolutely necessary for fetal development. Low zinc levels are linked to premature births, low birth weight, growth retardation, and preeclampsia (see chapter 2). Mercury can prevent zinc from doing its many important jobs in the body. So it is important to have enough zinc in the diet, especially if you are exposed to mercury. Zinc can be found in high amounts in oysters, other shellfish, fish, and red meats. Good amounts are found in plant foods such as whole grains, legumes, nuts, and seeds. Since zinc competes with calcium and iron for absorption into the body, it's a good idea to take it separately from these other minerals.

Calcium

We know that mercury causes problems in the function of the brain and nerves. To function properly, nerves use calcium. Mercury prevents calcium from being used by nerve cells and can cause the cells to die. Other studies show that mercury (and lead) can cause blood vessels to contract or squeeze shut by interfering with calcium levels in the cells that make up the vessel walls. This causes high blood pressure that may damage the heart.

Magnesium

Magnesium is a mineral that is essential for the body's formation of energy from food. It is needed to make ATP (adenosine triphosphate), the compound that stores energy and delivers it where needed in the body. This energy is needed for nerves to work, for muscles to contract, for our bodies to use sugar properly, and for hundreds of other reactions in the body. Mercury can stop or reduce many of these reactions that use magnesium. It does this by fooling body systems into thinking it is magnesium. When the body tries to use the mercury for its reactions, it doesn't work. These reactions are those for nerve and muscle function, heart muscle and blood vessel function, bone structure (with calcium), brain function, and sugar metabolism.

Vitamin E

Vitamin E (tocopherol) is a vitamin with strong antioxidant properties. This means that it helps the body detoxify harmful chemicals and also protects cells in the body from being destroyed by toxic substances. Studies show that vitamin E can reduce the toxic effects of mercury. It protects the genetic material (DNA) in the cells and also the reproductive cells from the toxic effects of mercury. Vitamin E also prevents the premature rupture of membranes during pregnancy, thus preventing premature birth.

Fiber

Fiber can reduce the absorption of toxins such as mercury into the body. This is especially true of water-soluble fiber such as is found in vegetables, pears, apples, legumes, powdered psyllium seed husks, guar gum, pectin, and oat bran. The fiber binds to the toxins in the digestive tract and helps them exit the body more quickly.

See Appendixes for lists of foods containing the above nutrients.

The Politics Behind Mercury

If one thing is true, it's that large, powerful organizations or institutions don't like change—especially if such change is going to cost them large sums of money. An example is the B vitamin folic acid. Research showing that it decreases the risk of birth defects has been available for over 30 years. But it was just recently, in 1999, that the U.S. government came out and said that foods should be fortified with folic acid and could contain labels stating that folic acid decreases the risk of birth defects. The American Dental Association, the 800-pound gorilla of the dental world, doesn't like change either. They approved of mercury amalgams for 150 years and are not about to shift gears, whatever the evidence. That this is true can best be seen in the *60 Minutes* interview with Morley Safer.

In 1986, the ADA changed its code of ethics to make it a violation of that code for any dentist to recommend the removal of amalgam because of the mercury. Dr. Joel Berger, a dentist who was removing amalgams, was charged with fraud by the New York State dental authorities. The ADA provided an expert witness to testify against him. His license was revoked. Dr. Berger never told a patient that they would get healthier or better from a disease if he removed mercury amalgams. He just told them that he could remove a known risk, a poison, toxin, and carcinogen from their bodies. Dr. Murray Vimy of the World Health Organization testified as a scientific expert in Berger's defense. Dr. Vimy said that the United States has taken away the constitutional rights of dentists and the rights of patients who no longer have freedom of choice or expression. "A dentist can no longer say he is against dental amalgam, so it's a fear tactic. It's a witch hunt," said Dr. Vimy.

The ADA representative, Dr. Heber Simmons, denied that it was a witch hunt and said that evidence that removing amalgams helps disease is just anecdotal. The word *anecdotal* doesn't mean a report is not true. It means that a doctor has observed a change in a patient, or a few patients, but a large-scale scientific study has not yet been done. For example, Dr. Alfred Zamm, an allergist and dermatologist in Kingston, New York, reported that hundreds of his patients recovered from a variety of diseases including arthritis and allergies after having fillings removed. While Dr. Simmons didn't totally dismiss the anecdotal evidence he felt that the facts were "clinically insignificant," and said that there were only 50 cases of amalgam allergy reported in the previous 85 years. The point that he missed, however, is that we are not talking about allergies. Says Dr. Zamm, "It's not allergy. It's poisoning of the critical immune processes." Even if the problem is allergy to mercury, why aren't patients tested for mercury allergy before fillings are put into their teeth?

Morley Safer then asked, "If the mercury in amalgam fillings is as poisonous as you say it is, why hasn't the medical community jumped on it and banned it?" Dr. Zamm said that diagnosing mercury poisoning is difficult because each affected person may have different symptoms: tiredness in one person, headaches in another, joint pain in someone else. Also, doctors are unfamiliar with the disease and its symptoms.

In the United States, a ban on mercury amalgams would have to come from the FDA. The FDA says that while research raises some preliminary questions about the safety of dental amalgams, more research has to be done. The FDA is confident in the value of amalgams in dental care and won't ban them until it is satisfied that there is a health risk. However, according to Dr. Vimy, the FDA's dental division consists mostly of people from the American Dental Association and the dental materials industry. There is virtually no medical or scientific input and so, "anything the ADA wants, they pretty much can get through the FDA," says Dr. Vimy. While the ADA's Dr. Simmons says that there "absolutely" is scientific evidence that mercury amalgam is safe, the ADA's top scientist (who was present at the interview) says the effects of mercury vapor on health have not yet been well researched. They contradict each other.

Right now, patients don't have the right to know about what goes into their mouths. With any prescription drug, you are entitled to give "informed consent" before you take it. This means that you were told about the good and the bad effects of the drug. But the ADA is fighting any legislation that would make dentists have to explain the risks of amalgams to their patients. Safer asked Dr. Simmons whether he tells patients about the controversy. When Safer said it sounded like the ADA doesn't want him or other dentists to volunteer information to patients, Simmons slipped and said, "Oh no, I'm not volunteering. I mean, I'm not saying that." Simmons said he would only tell patients if they asked. *How can you ask a question if you don't know there is a problem?* Of course, after reading this chapter you know what to ask and what to do. Please tell everyone you know and care about the facts on mercury!

Money counts. Dr. Vimy went on to say that if you took amalgam off the market, about 40% of American dentists who belong to the ADA would have to go back to school to learn how to use other substances besides mercury amalgam to fill teeth. These dentists would lose a lot of money while being trained. Said Dr. Zamm, "If it's not reasonably safe, if there's a question, I'm not going to put it in my child's mouth." So much for politics. The FDA is still reviewing the safety of amalgam fillings. Nothing has changed—except that now you know what is going on!

More Mercury in the Environment

The National Academy of Sciences is now doing a study to find out what the toxic effects of mercury are and whether the Environmental Protection Agency has properly set the minimum toxic dose. Mercury in the environment comes from coal-burning power plants, incinerators, mining, and other sources. The mercury in the air rains down into rivers, lakes, and the ocean where it is converted by bacteria into the very toxic methyl mercury. This form of mercury is taken up and stored in the fatty tissues of fish. The concentrations of mercury are increasing: airborne mercury is about three to six times the level it was in preindustrial times. Studies have shown that mercury exposure can lead to subtle effects such as reduced coordination and vision problems.

Alternatives to Toxic Fillings

When you choose a dentist for your child (or for yourself) you should ask the following question: "Do you place mercury fillings?" A dentist that says "yes" may not have enough experience using nonmetal filling material. If the dentist tells you that mercury will not cause any problems, look for another dentist. It is probably not worth the effort to try to educate the dentist about the toxicity of mercury. Look for a dentist who has experience in using nonmercury filling material. There are other substances that can be used to fill and repair teeth besides mercury-containing amalgams.

An article in the November 1998 *Journal of the American Den-*

tal Association noted (thank goodness!) that the use of mercury amalgam appears to be declining. Its use has dropped from 85% in 1988 to 58% in 1997. The article predicted that the use of mercury amalgam would continue to diminish and will eventually disappear from the scene. But this change is not due to any concern over mercury contamination of the human body. One reason is that there are new materials that are just as durable and strong and, unlike silver-colored fillings, can be made to match the color of a patient's teeth. Because their teeth look better, more patients are asking for the new materials. Although these materials—composites, glass ionomers, and metal-ceramic crowns—are not toxic like mercury, they are more costly. The cost is from 1.5 times to 8 times the cost of mercury amalgam fillings. However, paying more now will prevent you and your child from really paying (with your health) later.

In one study, filling material called resin-modified glass ionomer cement was compared to mercury-containing amalgam. The researchers checked the fillings at 6-month, 1-year, 2-year, and 3-year dentist appointments. The results showed no significant differences between the resin-modified glass ionomer cement fillings and the amalgam restorations. The resin-modified glass ionomer cement worked just as well as amalgam for filling teeth. In fact, the resin-modified glass ionomer showed significantly less damage from caries to the enamel of the tooth where the filling material touched it than did amalgam.

Gallium is a metal that is substituted for mercury in an amalgam-like alloy (called galloy). It looks and behaves like the traditional mercury-containing amalgam. Gallium, however, has minimal allergy and toxicity potential according to scientific literature. Before it was put on the market, studies showed that if galloy is placed in the tooth with meticulous care, it will function acceptably. However, galloy placed without proper sealing and with moisture contamination has caused sensitivity and/or tooth fracture. Sealing is recommended by the manufacturer and must be done before galloy placement and after carving (shaping) the filling in order to prevent moisture contamination during early use. So galloy can provide mercury-free metallic restoration of teeth.

In 1997, Colorado Governor Roy Romer signed into law a bill to increase Colorado residents' access to mercury-free dentistry. Called the Colorado Dental Freedom Law, it was created to give consumers the right to choose safe, effective alternatives to mercury amalgam fillings. The law, the first of its kind in the United States, lets patients choose mercury-free dentistry from dentists licensed in the state. It also ensures that the dentists can continue to practice mercury-free dentistry without facing legal action.

CHAPTER 12

Orthodontics: Making the Right Choice for Your Child

In earlier chapters, we've given you lots of important preventive information, so you can avoid orthodontic problems. We've talked about diet before and during pregnancy, the importance of breast feeding, and the use of the correct nipple and pacifier.

However, if you already have children with problems that need to be corrected with orthodontic treatment, we want to help you be aware of certain things before you begin treatment, as there are options your dentist may not know, or may not tell you.

What Is Orthodontics?

Orthodontics is the branch of dentistry that specializes in preventing and treating dental and facial problems. The technical term for these problems is *malocclusion,* which means "bad bite." We often think of orthodontics as just the straightening of teeth, but it is much more. All orthodontists are dentists, but only about 6% of dentists are orthodontists. An orthodontist must first go to college and then complete a 4-year dental graduate program at a university dental school or other institution accredited by the Commission on Dental Accreditation of the American Dental Association. The dentist must then successfully complete an additional 2- to 3-year residency program of advanced education in orthodontics. The ADA must also accredit this residency program. Only dentists who have successfully completed this advanced specialty education may call themselves orthodontists.

Orthodontics requires a dentist to have skill in the design and use of corrective "appliances," such as braces, to bring teeth, lips, and jaws into proper alignment so that there will be facial balance. Just as important, as you will see, is making sure the tongue is doing its job in helping the teeth align properly.

We know from personal experience, and from friends and relatives, that orthodontic work can be expensive and uncomfortable for your child and that it may take a long time to complete. It would be nice to avoid it or get it over with more quickly. We will try to help you achieve this objective.

We talked earlier about the importance of breast feeding in helping to properly develop your baby's jaws, face, and teeth. Breast-fed babies use their tongues and cheek muscles properly. Having straight teeth begins at the breast. The problems that come with an abnormal swallowing pattern and the wrong type of tongue movements were discussed in chapter 4. Dan Garliner, the speech therapist who developed the system of myofunctional therapy, said that 74% of orthodontic cases come from an abnormal swallow as a major cause. So by starting early with breast feeding rather than bottle feeding, or at least using the correct nipple, many orthodontic problems can be avoided or corrected more easily.

In this chapter, we'd like to add some more information on how to stop orthodontic work in its tracks. Braces really do look like tracks, something your child will be happier without. But if your child has or needs braces, we have some information that will help get you both through it.

Early Signs of Future Problems: Interceptive Orthodontics

Early treatment of orthodontic problems is called *interceptive orthodontics*. With this early treatment or *intervention,* it is less likely that permanent teeth will have to be removed. The final results are also more stable (do not revert) than waiting until growth is nearly complete when all the permanent teeth have grown in.

In many cases, the problems needing an orthodontist are inherited such as crowding of teeth, too much space between teeth, extra or missing teeth, and a wide variety of other irregularities of the jaws, teeth, and face. For example, you might inherit your mother's small jaw and your father's large teeth; if this were the case, your teeth would be too large to fit your jaw.

For others, the problems can be caused by thumb, finger, or pacifier sucking (with the wrong type of pacifier), airway blockage by tonsils and adenoids, dental disease, or premature loss of primary (baby) or permanent teeth. If you lose a tooth in an accident, the remaining teeth may start to drift into the empty space. You can lose a tooth early to cavities or gum disease; this often leaves a space that other teeth drift toward.

Whether inherited or not, many of these problems can affect facial development and appearance as well as the teeth. We'd like to catch the problems early, when it is easier to correct them.

Why is it important to prevent or treat orthodontic problems? First of all, crooked and crowded teeth are hard to clean. This may lead to tooth decay, gum disease, and eventually tooth loss. If front teeth stick out, they can be injured more easily. There can be increased wear, and poor chewing habits can put too much stress on gum tissue and the bone that supports the teeth. There can be interference with the normal growth and development of the jaws. The jaw joints may not function properly, which can cause chronic headaches or pain in the face or neck. Problems with swallowing can result from untreated orthodontic problems just as abnormal swallowing can cause orthodontic problems. If there are swallowing problems, facial muscles will not move properly and the features of the face can change as the child grows. Speech defects can be another effect of untreated orthodontic problems.

Don't wait to correct problems with a palate that needs to be widened. If your child gets interceptive orthodontic treatment at age 8, when the palate is growing rapidly, the treatment will be uncomfortable, but not tremendously painful. By the time your child is 12, the bones in the roof of the mouth will have hardened. Corrective work done at this time to expand the palate will be much more painful. If you wait until your child is 20 to do palatal expansion, it will entail major surgery to correct a palatal problem.

When left untreated, many orthodontic problems become worse. Preventive dentistry, like preventive medicine, as always is the best (and least expensive) choice.

What Should Parents Look For?

Peter Treyz, D.D.S., a dentist in Katonah, New York, for 40 years, looks for the early signs that would lead to orthodontic work if not corrected. He works with two general dentists and a myofunctional therapist, Patricia Stoddard. When children 6 or 7 years of age come in for a checkup, Dr. Treyz will look at the child's mouth first. If he thinks the child could use myofunctional therapy, he will work on this first before any attempt is made to use braces.

He uses myofunctional therapy for 80% of his patients (children as well as adults). "The sooner myofunctional therapy is done, the sooner the mouth starts to develop in a normal way," says Dr. Treyz. If the children do need braces at 10 or 11 years of age, Dr. Treyz does not have to extract as many teeth as other dentists do. He rarely takes out permanent teeth; maybe three or four patients (less than 1%) a year get extractions. With myofunctional therapy first, there is less chance that permanent teeth will have to come out.

The Mittelmans feel that it is absolutely essential for a child with an abnormal swallow to have myofunctional therapy before having orthodontia. They have observed that:

- After myofunctional therapy, the teeth often move to a more normal position, lessening the amount of orthodontic treatment needed.
- If orthodontia is done without first doing myofunctional therapy, it can take longer, be more difficult, and not produce as good a result.
- An abnormal swallow, if left untreated, can cause orthodontic treatment to relapse, that is, the teeth can shift back to their original position. Or, a retainer may be needed indefinitely to maintain the orthodontic correction.

How can parents tell whether their child is having a problem with an abnormal swallow or other problems that would need myofunctional therapy? Here are some things to look for, according to Dr. Treyz:

- Thumb sucking or other oral habits such as sucking other fingers or blankets
- Talking with a lisp, which happens when the middle part of the tongue doesn't move properly
- An inability to eat dry foods easily; the child needs to wash dry food down with liquids
- Chronic stomach problems, which may be caused by problems with chewing and swallowing
- Mouth breathing; if the mouth gets dry from being open, the child can get inflammation of the tonsils, chronic sore throat, and cracking around the mouth
- A higher incidence of allergies; when the mouth is open all the time, the tiny hairs that line the airways can't work to push out airborne allergens, which can then get down into the lungs faster, as can cold air, another irritant

Other early signs include:

- Early or late loss of baby teeth
- Difficulty in chewing or biting
- Crowding, misplaced, or blocked-out teeth
- Jaws that shift or make sounds
- Biting the cheek or roof of the mouth
- Teeth that meet abnormally or not at all
- Jaws and teeth that are out of proportion to the rest of the face

Your child's doctor may see an allergy problem or treat your child for chronic stomach aches, but the dentist usually does not hear about these problems. These two health professionals don't talk to each other, so neither one is getting the whole picture. "The dentists of today should be holistic—they should be the doctors of the mouth," says Dr. Treyz. This means that the dentist should understand what he or she sees in the mouth. The mouth is really the window of the body; many problems in other parts of the body start or can be seen in the mouth. For example, beside allergies, vitamin deficiencies can show up in the mouth. A deficiency in B vitamins can cause a shiny tongue and cracks in the lips. Even a mild vitamin C deficiency can cause bleeding gums. A holistic dentist will look at the tongue, teeth, cheeks, adenoids, and tonsils—the whole picture.

What Are the Benefits of Early Treatment?

When there are signs that a child should have early orthodontic treatment, getting this treatment can be very beneficial because it can:

- guide the proper growth of the jaw
- regulate the width of the upper and lower dental arches (the arch-shaped jawbone that supports the teeth), so that teeth will meet properly
- ensure that new permanent teeth grow in the correct positions
- decrease the risk of accidents that may happen to upper front teeth that may stick out
- correct harmful oral habits such as thumb or finger sucking
- reduce or eliminate abnormal swallowing or speech problems
- improve personal appearance and self-esteem
- shorten the treatment time for braces if needed later
- reduce the likelihood of impacted permanent teeth (teeth that should have come in, but have not), and
- preserve or gain space for permanent teeth that are coming in

One situation where early treatment is very beneficial is when a tooth falls out early. An accident or dental disease may cause the tooth loss. Baby teeth are important; they help normal development of the jawbones and muscles, save space for the permanent teeth, and guide them into correct positions. Some baby teeth are not replaced by permanent teeth until the child is 12 or 14 years old. So it is never a good idea to leave the problem alone. A space maintainer can help avoid future problems. Space maintainers are made of metal or plastic and are custom fitted to your child's mouth. They are small, and most children adjust to them after the first few days. Keeping the space for the permanent tooth prevents more expensive orthodontic treatment later. Teeth next to the gap may tilt or drift into the space. Teeth in the other half of the jaw may move up or down to fill the gap left by the lost tooth.

As with braces, children should avoid sticky sweets or chewing gum when a spacer is in the mouth. Tell your child not to push on or tug at the space maintainer with fingers or tongue. Keep the spacer clean, brush and floss, and continue regular dentist visits.

What Are the Most Commonly Treated Orthodontic Problems?

There are a number of conditions that can be corrected with orthodontics. Here are some of the most familiar:

Crowding: If not treated, there may be impacted teeth, poor biting relationships, and an undesirable appearance.

Overjet or protruding upper teeth: Unlike overbite, which refers to when the upper incisor teeth overlap the lower ones, overjet refers to when the upper teeth stick out too far into the lips, which make these teeth easy to injure. This often indicates poor bite of the back teeth (molars) and may indicate unevenness in jaw growth such as a short lower jaw. Thumb- and finger-sucking habits can also cause a protrusion of the upper front teeth.

Open bite: This means that the upper and lower front (incisor) teeth do not touch when biting down. This open space between the upper and lower front teeth causes all the chewing pressure to be placed on the back teeth. This excessive biting pressure and rubbing together of the back teeth makes it difficult for the child to chew and may cause much wearing down of the teeth.

Spacing: If teeth are missing or small, or the dental arch is very wide, there can be space between the teeth. The more space between the teeth, the less attractive the mouth will look.

Crossbite: This is when the upper teeth bite inside the lower teeth (toward the tongue). Crossbites of both back teeth and front teeth need to be corrected early because they cause biting and chewing problems.

Underbite or lower jaw protrusion: About 3% to 5% of people have a lower jaw that is longer than the upper jaw. This can cause the lower front teeth to stick out ahead of the upper front teeth, creating a crossbite. As the jaw grows and the teeth develop, this condition needs to be watched and corrected if necessary.

Braces, Wires, and Waiting

Before we talk about orthodontic work, you may want to know how braces can move teeth that have roots that seem to be attached to the skull. We know that when a baby tooth is lost too early or when there is an extraction of a permanent tooth, the teeth around the space can shift position by tilting. Or the whole tooth may shift in one direction or another. These are examples of tooth movement. This movement is possible because the teeth are not stuck in the jawbone. Teeth, as we discussed earlier, are actually attached to the bone with a type of connective tissue called the periodontal ligament. We explained how taking care of the gums and good nutrition could keep this ligament strong and healthy and able to keep the teeth from falling out.

Inside the bone are certain cells that help bone form and break down. The cells that lay down new bone are called *osteoblasts,* while those that remove old bone are called *osteoclasts.* Bone, you see, is not a dead substance. It is filled with cells that are constantly working and using nutrients to do their work.

Braces work by slowly putting pressure on the tooth. The tooth, in turn, presses on the bone. Where there is pressure, the osteoclasts remove the bone so that the tooth can move in that direction. When the tooth moves, the space left behind it is filled in by the osteoblasts. This can take time and explains why orthodontic work takes so long. If it is done too quickly, the roots of the teeth can dissolve in the body's effort to let the tooth move faster.

There is, alas, no "quick fix" for crooked teeth. You can also see why calcium and other minerals are important for the teeth and bones, which are always remodeling.

How Orthodontic Work Is Done

The usual types of braces that you see are those that are fixed in the child's mouth until the orthodontic work is finished. Braces can also be removable. These are made of wires and plastic. Some fit the upper and lower teeth at the same time. An advantage of this type is that it is easier to keep clean. The braces can be taken out whenever needed.

However, the problem with removable braces is getting children to keep them in their mouths. For success with removable braces your child must wear them exactly as instructed by the orthodontist. So that is why most dentists used fixed, or nonremovable, braces.

In many cases, children are given braces when there really isn't much of a problem with the alignment of the teeth. People of all ages with minor problems just want treatment because "everyone should get their teeth straightened." This is okay as long as a family can afford the work, assuming that good orthodontic treatment is given. That's not always the case. Front teeth so nicely straightened can revert back to crookedness because the jawbone is too small.

Not correcting the abnormal swallow is also a reason for retainers being used over and over again. When the child has braces, and the work is completed, the teeth will get out of line again if the tongue keeps pushing on them. This causes the bite to shift and a retainer is again needed. It's too bad that this matter of abnormal swallow is almost totally ignored in dental school, much like the dangers of mercury. Ask your dentist or orthodontist about it to see how well informed he or she is about the subject. Unfortunately, most dentists are unaware of the details behind the controversy.

There are other problems and side effects. Perfectly good back teeth are often removed to make room for lining up the front teeth. The result may be nice straight front teeth, but looking at the face from the side, many of these children can have very flat or nearly concave profiles and weak lips. Too much extra space is often created, leaving annoying spaces between the teeth.

When braces move teeth, the roots of the teeth may start to dissolve, leaving the teeth weak in their bony sockets. This happens in as many as one out of eight orthodontic patients. The gums can also shrink from tooth movement or poorly fitted bands.

In general, active treatment time with braces can take from 1 to 3 years. Interceptive, or early treatment, procedures may take only a few months. The actual time depends on the growth of the child's mouth and face, how well the child (and parents) cooperates, and how severe the problem was to begin with. Some children will respond faster to treatment than others will.

We hope that a combination of breast feeding, good oral habits, good nutrition, and correction of tongue problems can help you and your child avoid a long and expensive course of orthodontic treatment. This may not be the case since there are some things we can't do anything about, such as inherited problems and when you start using our advice. So we'd like to give you some more information about braces to help you make decisions about what goes into your child's mouth.

Braces are custom made for your child by the orthodontist according to the problem being treated. As we said above, they may be removable or fixed to the teeth by cement. They may be made of metal, ceramic, or plastic. The braces are adjusted to put a constant, gentle force on the teeth in the right direction. Over time the braces can slowly move the teeth through their supporting bone to a new position.

After braces are first put on there is usually some discomfort. There is also discomfort when the braces are adjusted during treatment. Right after braces are put on, the teeth may feel sore and tender when your child bites and chews. This can last from 3 to 5 days. Natural pain remedies can help, especially those that can be rubbed on the teeth and gums. The lips, cheeks, and tongue may also be irritated for 1 to 2 weeks. After that, they will toughen and become used to the braces. In some cases, wearing braces will affect a child's speech. However, this is usually temporary. Most children can speak clearly in a day or two. The child with braces can safely run, jump, swim, and play.

Other Kinds of Appliances

There are other "helper" appliances used with braces that may shorten the time needed to complete orthodontic work and that are used for special problems. These may include headgear, a bionator, the Herbst appliance, and maxillary expansion appliance. These are removable appliances, made of plastic and wires, which fit the upper teeth, and sometimes the roof of the mouth. They resemble an orthodontic retainer worn after completion of orthodontic treatment. An exception is the head gear (or night brace) that has a band going around the head. They are used to guide the growth and development of jaws in children or teenagers.

For example, an upper jaw expansion appliance can dramatically widen a narrow upper jaw in a few months. This appliance has a spring in the palatal portion that exerts force on the upper teeth, pushing them outward. During treatment, a headgear or Herbst appliance, or an activator-type appliance such as a bionator, can dramatically reduce the protrusion (sticking out) of upper front teeth or retrusion (inward position) of the lower jaw (a lower jaw that is too far behind the upper jaw), while making upper and lower jaw lengths more equal. A bionator brings the upper and lower jaws into a different relationship in a way that induces the muscles of the lips, face and jaws to put pressure on groups of teeth. A headgear uses the force of a band around the top of the head or back of the neck to put backward pressure on upper front or back teeth.

The wires used today to attach one tooth to the next are less noticeable than earlier ones because they are thinner and not as shiny. Wires are no longer made only of stainless steel. They can be alloys (mixtures) of nickel, titanium, copper, and cobalt. Some of the wires are heat-activated. This means that the heat from the mouth causes the wire to move, gently pulling the teeth into line. The heat-activated wire made of a nickel-titanium alloy was made by the National Aeronautics and Space Agency (NASA) to automatically activate antennas or solar panels of spacecraft orbiting into the sun's rays. These new kinds of wires may reduce the number of appointments needed to make adjustments to the wires. A type of clear orthodontic wire is also being tested.

One question that is often asked is whether there are less noticeable braces. Braces used in the past had a metal band with a bracket (the part of the braces that hold the wire) put around each tooth. Now the front teeth usually have only the bracket bonded to the tooth.

Brackets can be made of metal, or can be clear or colored, depending on your choice.

In some cases, brackets may be bonded behind the teeth (called lingual braces). Lingual braces used to be in fashion, but they are rarely used today, and only when a patient insists that the braces absolutely cannot show. Lingual braces are much more uncomfortable than standard braces. The orthodontic treatment is much more painful, and the treatment takes almost twice as long. There is also difficulty in talking normally with lingual braces.

Not Worth a Nickel

We believe that there is no place for the use of nickel in the mouth. Author Hal Huggins, D.D.S., had this to say about nickel: "Nickel is one of the most durable yet most carcinogenic (cancer-causing) metals on this planet. . . . As far as nickel being carcinogenic is concerned, that has been published in the scientific literature for over fifty years. Animal studies demonstrating malignancies as a result of exposure to nickel have been shown in multiple strains of rats, mice, guinea pigs, rabbits, and cats."

Care of Teeth With Braces

Teeth with braces need special care. Your child must be careful to avoid hard foods since they can bend the wires, loosen the bands, or break the brackets. Fruits and vegetables should be cut up into smaller pieces and chewed with the back teeth. Sticky foods such as gum, raisins, toffee, and caramel can also bend and break the wires and brackets. It's particularly important to avoid foods containing sugar, since the teeth cannot be cleaned as well in areas blocked by brackets and wires.

Your child should not chew on pens, pencils, or fingernails because chewing on hard things can damage the braces. If braces are damaged by accidental falls or in sports, treatment will take longer, requiring extra trips to the orthodontist's office.

Keeping the teeth and braces clean is very important. Mouth hygiene with braces in place takes more skill and more time than for a mouth without braces. A good cleaning must be done every day if the teeth and gums are to be healthy during and after orthodontic treatment. Children who do not keep their teeth clean may have to see the dentist more often for professional cleaning.

The orthodontist and staff will teach you and your child how to care for the teeth, gums, and braces during treatment. This teaching will include how often to brush and how often to floss.

Flossing with braces takes longer than without them. Your child should use a soft toothbrush or a special orthodontic toothbrush with bristles that can clean around the braces (see Resources). Floss threaders can help with flossing.

The orthodontist may suggest other cleaning aids that might help your child maintain good dental health. For example, an interdental brush can fit between the wire and the tooth to remove hard-to-reach plaque and food particles. Water irrigators can be used along with brushing and flossing. This helps remove food particles and plaque.

To keep teeth and gums healthy, you must continue with regular visits to the family dentist during orthodontic treatment. It's also very important for your child to cooperate during what may be a long, uncomfortable treatment. Your child must carefully clean his or her teeth, may have to wear rubber bands, headgear, or other appliances as prescribed by the orthodontist, and will have to keep appointments as scheduled.

After the braces are removed, a retainer may be used to hold the teeth in their new position until they are stable. Retainers are often worn for several hours a day or during sleep.

Temporomandibular joint (TMJ) disorder

One of the problems associated with abnormal swallow patterns is temporomandibular joint (TMJ) disorder. The TMJ is located where the jaw meets the skull bone just in front of the ear. TMJ problems can cause pain, headache, and cracking noises when there is jaw movement. Just doing orthodontic work without correcting abnormal swallow will result in the TMJ remaining a problem or it will come back again. In some cases, correcting the abnormal swallow using myofunctional therapy will prevent the development of TMJ disorder. When the tongue presses on the teeth during the act of swallowing instead of pressing on the hard palate in the roof of the mouth as it should, teeth get out of line. The tongue actually acts like a brace pushing against the teeth, and the teeth will move.

At first, the slight movement of the teeth caused by the pressing tongue won't be noticeable. However, soon the upper and lower teeth will interfere with one another when the jaws open and shut. When the jaw shifts the joints also shift, and this triggers the TMJ disorder. Abnormal swallowing can also make the TMJ disorder worse if it's already present. It can also cause teeth grinding. The body tries to wear down the teeth that are rubbing together and find a comfortable place for them to rest.

However, this brings only temporary relief. Even orthodontic work to align the teeth may not prevent TMJ disorder from returning. Unless the tongue movement is made normal, the TMJ problems will keep coming back.

When we (Jerome and Beverly) were practicing dentistry, a girl came to us for pain in her TMJs. We adjusted the biting surfaces of certain teeth, and she did very well; her TMJ pain was relieved. However, in 3 months she returned with the same symptoms. We again relieved the irregular bite. Again she showed great improvement and relief from her symptoms. She was distressed, as we were, when her pain returned several months later. Soon after that we began to understand the importance of the abnormal swallow, so we started using myofunctional therapy. We found that the girl had an abnormal swallow. When she swallowed, her tongue pressed against her lower right teeth just in front of the back molars.

We explained to her that relieving her bite helped only temporarily because her tongue continually pressed against these teeth. We suggested that if she could have this harmful swallowing pattern corrected, her TMJ symptoms would be treated more successfully. She worked hard and was eager to correct her abnormal swallow. When we were sure that she was swallowing correctly, we equilibrated (balanced) the biting surfaces of her teeth once more.

When we checked after several years, she still had no symptoms. We see many similar problems that could have been prevented. The TMJ syndrome is most often caused by bite irregularities. We see these irregularities when the upper and lower teeth do not come together harmoniously when the jaw closes. The brain must send messages to the closing muscles to jiggle and twist the jaw in an attempt to bring the teeth together tightly.

Many of our TMJ patients previously had orthodontic treatment. In these cases, the teeth were moved into new positions.

Moving the teeth changes the bite, which can cause traumatic occlusion and the TMJ dysfunction disorder. This makes it necessary to adjust the biting surfaces of the teeth to put the upper and lower teeth into a properly balanced relationship.

We call this *occlusal equilibration*. Neglecting this step can, and often does, result in the patient's developing the TMJ disorder. Unfortunately, few dentists know much about occlusal equilibration, and so this is a much neglected area in dental care.

How to Find a Good Orthodontist

We would recommend that you ask your general dentist for names of orthodontists—assuming that you have a general dentist who has the same ideas about dental treatment as you have.

Many dentists and pedodontists (children's dentists) who are concerned about prevention do interceptive orthodontia. By law, dentists who practice orthodontia do not have to be board certified.

There are dentists that are more supportive of doing removable appliance therapy, and avoiding the extraction of teeth for orthodontic treatment, than other orthodontists. Some of the supportive dentists belong to the American Association for the Study of Orthodontics (see Resources). Getting the best orthodontic treatment for your child may mean considering an experienced dentist who is not a board-certified orthodontist.

The next step would be to call the orthodontist's office. There are some questions that you might want to ask on the telephone. Talk to the orthodontist's assistant about the methods the orthodontist uses and his or her general treatment philosophy. Find out how the orthodontist deals with pain, how long treatment usually lasts, and what it costs. You do need to shop around, because charges can be very different from one office to the next. You may not get all the answers, but it's worth asking. We hope that our information can help you decide which dentist is the right one to treat your child.

Used Braces—You Put What in My Child's Mouth?

There are other very important questions to ask the orthodontist *before* you start treatment. Does he or she recycle the materials from one patient's mouth to another? That's right! Many orthodontists will use the metal materials—braces, brackets and so on—on the next patient. Brackets are removed from one patient's mouth, sent out for cleaning, and then bonded into another patient's mouth. As many as one in three U.S. orthodontists will reuse some materials from one patient's mouth to the next patient's mouth.

Reuse of orthodontic materials is an ongoing problem, but whether this is safe is still not clear. There is no guarantee that sterilization procedures will kill all germs—and this is assuming that the sterilization is done correctly in the first place. Reused materials may also work less effectively because they are worn down from use.

Ask about the sterilization procedures used in the orthodontist's office. Orthodontic materials can be sterilized in dry heat sterilizers, autoclaves, or a solution called glutaraldehyde. When used properly, dry heat sterilizers and autoclaves kill all known infectious agents. The glutaraldehyde solution does not always kill the AIDS virus. Therefore, although the chances of your child's catching AIDS in the orthodontist's office are very low, you should make sure that the orthodontist uses an autoclave or dry heat sterilizer on all of his instruments. If glutaraldehyde solution is used, find another orthodontist. There are no governmental guidelines that prevent the use of "recycled" orthodontic materials in the United States, although this practice is prohibited in Europe.

You should also make sure that everyone in the office who works on your child—the orthodontist and any staff—wears gloves and changes the gloves before each patient. Washing the gloves is not good enough. If they do not use fresh gloves, find another orthodontic office. You may also want to ask if new materials such as wires are sterilized before being put in your child's mouth. Although the materials may be sterilized at the factory where they are made, there is no guarantee that they are still sterile when it's time to use them.

In 1988, the Centers for Disease Control and the American Dental Association issued new sterilization guidelines and sterilizer standards because of the AIDS epidemic. Parts of the guideline were formally adopted by the American Association for Medical Instruments in 1996. On August 14, 1998, the FDA formally accepted the standard and published it in the *Code of Federal Regulations*. Unfortunately, not every orthodontist is aware of, or follows, all of the guidelines.

Is there anything else you can do to prevent your child from getting used orthodontic materials? If you have already chosen an orthodontist, talk to him or her about your concerns. Most orthodontists will not use materials that have already been used in a previous patient's mouth without your consent. If you found out later that such materials were being used, and you had not signed a consent form, this would be grounds for a lawsuit. So any reputable orthodontist will ask for your consent. Read carefully any consent forms that your orthodontist asks you to sign.

Of course, the reason for using recycled materials is to save money. If you belong to a managed care plan with a dental benefit, it's a good bet that the orthodontists belonging to that plan are recycling. Many of these plans are priced low because they assume that the orthodontist will not have to buy any new orthodontic materials for your child. If you have such a dental plan, talk with the plan administrator to make sure that the orthodontists they contract with use only fresh materials in your child's mouth. This may be difficult to ensure. If your plan administrator will not pay for fresh materials for your child, then talk to your orthodontist about paying for your orthodontic materials yourself. Some orthodontists will let you do this.

Allergies to Orthodontic Materials

Braces may cause soreness of the gums and mouth at first. However, if your child continues to hurt, it could be a sign that he or she is allergic to something in the braces. Your orthodontist can check for this. Your child's mouth will also be sore if he or she is not doing a good job of brushing and flossing. If dental hygiene is good, then you should consider allergies.

If a child is allergic to begin with, you should discuss your child's allergies with your orthodontist. You will want to make sure that your child is not allergic to something in the orthodontist's office, or allergic to the orthodontic materials.

There are usually two kinds of allergies to orthodontic products: allergies to the metals used, such as nickel, chrome, and copper, and allergies to latex. Metal allergies are fairly common, but generally not very serious. The symptoms are an inflammation of the mouth and possibly inflammation at places on the body where metal (such as a watchband or ring) comes in contact with your child's skin. There may be sores in the mouth, a burning mouth, or whole-body reactions such as dermatitis (rash and/or itchy skin). Other symptoms include fatigue, headache, and malaise (feeling sickly). Metal allergies can develop during orthodontic treatment in a child who was not allergic before.

Latex allergy is less common but can be life-threatening. There are two kinds of latex allergies. The more common allergy, which is not very serious is actually a reaction to chemical additives used to make the latex product. This allergy causes a slight inflammation of the patient's mouth, but it goes away after the latex is removed. The other type of allergy, can be life-threatening. This allergy is a reaction to the latex itself and is quite similar to penicillin allergy. A person might be exposed to latex and have no symptoms for years. Then the person might break out in a rash. Thereafter, the patient is permanently sensitive to latex. He or she might break into hives and/or swelling in their face and hands perhaps 20 to 50 minutes after being exposed to latex in a rubber glove, for example. There is also latex in orthodontic rubber bands. Other patients have difficulty breathing. There can be several different symptoms. *If your child breaks out into hives soon after orthodontic rubber bands are changed, develops swelling in the hands or face, or has difficulty breathing, take the child directly to an urgent care facility or a hospital emergency room. Do not wait hoping that the symptoms will go away.*

If you know or suspect that your child has a latex allergy, ask your orthodontist to use only latex-free materials. Latex allergy gets worse with repeated exposure, and can lead to potentially fatal anaphylactic reactions.

A good orthodontist should be able to answer your questions about allergies. His staff should also be trained to recognize the symptoms of allergies.

In the Office: What Will the Orthodontist Do?

At the first visit, the orthodontist should take a past medical and dental history of your child. A thorough examination of the child's teeth, palate, and mouth should be done. Impressions of the teeth are taken and a plaster model is made so that the orthodontist can study it. It will also be used to compare later to see how the treatment is working. Photographs of the face and teeth may also be taken.

What about X-rays? X-rays are needed in order to determine what needs to be done. The orthodontist will usually do three sets of X-rays: *cephalometric* X-rays of the entire head showing the relationship of the teeth and jaws to the face and skull; *panoramic* X-rays, which show all upper and lower teeth in biting position and any teeth still developing within the jaws; and *bite-wing* X-rays of the upper and lower back teeth, which are taken by having the patient bite down on the X–ray film to hold it in place. The panoramic X-ray and the cephalometric X-rays allow the orthodontist to look for weaknesses in the jaw or any shallow roots, so that your child can avoid a painful TMJ problem or other difficulty later on. The bite-wing X-rays look for caries (cavities). If your child has a cavity under his or her braces, the cavity may get large during orthodontic treatment, and your child may get a toothache. The X-rays are needed to make sure that the treatment proceeds smoothly, with no unexpected complications.

Can anything be done to decrease your child's exposure to X-rays? There are X-ray shields that can help lower the X-ray exposure. The shield can be attached to the orthodontist's X-ray machine. It narrows the beam of the X-rays so the X-rays shine only on your child's teeth gums and cheeks and not elsewhere on the face or body. If your orthodontist does not have such a shield, you may want to ask about it. The American Association of Pediatric Dentistry maintains a page on X-ray use and safety.

Make sure the dentist uses a lead apron over the child's body— one that has an extension to cover the thyroid area in the neck. Also, be sure to give the child extra antioxidant nutritional supplements (vitamins C, E, and beta-carotene) before X-rays are taken to help the child's body handle the free radicals produced by the X-rays.

You can see from the above information that orthodontic work on your child is a treatment that you cannot walk into without being armed with information. If you know the right questions to ask, your child will have a much better chance of getting the proper care.

Summary

Children born in the year 2001 will live longer than ever. For a boy, the average age is 73 years and is almost 80 years for a girl. This is double the life expectancy of a newborn in 1900. Although new dental technologies will help these children of the millennium keep their teeth longer and looking better, there is still no substitute for some of the things we have talked about in this book:

- Good health of both the mother and father before conception
- A healthy diet before conception and during pregnancy and nursing
- Breast feeding your baby
- Good oral habits and excellent dental hygiene
- Limiting sweets and providing the best diet for your child
- Going regularly to a dentist who understands that good health and avoidance of toxic substances produces healthy children with good teeth
- Knowing the facts about mercury fillings and fluoride treatment
- Making the right choices about dental work and orthodontics

We have done our best, using our combined years of experience and knowledge to give you the facts—the truth and the plan that will give your child a healthy body and a beautiful smile. The next step is for you to put this information into practice. You are the only one who can give such a gift to your child, and we are happy that we could help!

Nutritious Foods for Expectant Mothers

- Three-bean salad with virgin olive oil marinade
- One half papaya filled with nonfat organic yogurt
- One half cantaloupe filled with chicken salad or low-fat cottage cheese
- Toasted whole-wheat pocket bread topped with pizza sauce, Italian seasoning, and mozzarella cheese (cook in broiler)
- Air-popped popcorn served with fruit juice and carbonated water
- Crunchy raw vegetables (carrots, celery, zucchini, broccoli) dunked in herb-seasoned, lowfat yogurt dip
- Peanut butter spread on a whole-wheat bagel and topped with raisins or banana slices
- Fat-free or low-fat milk, fresh fruit (frozen), and frozen orange juice concentrate mixed in a blender
- Corn tortillas cut into triangles, baked until crisp, and served with salsa and a glass of orange juice

Some Fluoride Facts

"The 'optimal' level of fluoride intake has NEVER been determined scientifically" (quote from the *Journal of the American Dental Association,* vol. 126, p. 625, Dec. 1995).

In 1993, the U.S. Department of Health and Human Services stated in its *Toxicological Profile on Fluoride,* "Existing data indicates that subsets of the population may be unusually susceptible to the toxic effects of fluoride and its compounds. These populations include the elderly, people with deficiencies of calcium, magnesium, and/or vitamin C, and people with cardiovascular and kidney problems."

Fluoride has never passed the controlled studies necessary for FDA approval as either a supplement or an additive to municipal water. All other drugs must receive this approval before they can be sold to the public. From *Fluoridation: The Overdosing of America.* International Center for Nutrition Research. *www.icnr.com).*

"Drinking water containing as little as 1.2 ppm fluoride will cause developmental disturbances. In light of our present knowledge of the subject, the potentialities for harm outweigh those for good" (statement by the American Dental Association in the *Journal of the American Dental Association,* October 1, 1944).

"When fluoride reaches the cells which make the enamel, it destroys them. The enamel laid down is irregular, mottled, porous and thin. As the poisoning worsens, the enamel may even be absent" (J. A. Albright, The Effect of Fluoride on the Mechanical Properties of Bone, *Transactions of the Annual Meeting of the Orthopedics Research Society,* pp. 3, 98, 1978).

Fluoride has a strong affinity for magnesium, calcium, and manganese and inactivates cellular function by making these minerals unavailable; ". . . evidence for the absence of a systemic anticaries effect of fluoride is now recognized by leading dental researchers" (statement in the *Journal of Dental Research,* vol. 69, Special Issue, 1990).

In a New Zealand study of 60,000 schoolchildren, it was found that fluoridation had no significant effect on the decay of permanent teeth (J. Colquhoun, *Community Dentistry and Epidemiology* 13:37–41, 1985).

In the largest study on fluoridation and tooth decay conducted by the U.S. Public Health Service on over 39,000 schoolchildren, the decay rate of permanent teeth was virtually the same for fluoridated and nonfluoridated areas (W. Marcus, *Chemical and Engineering News,* 1990).

Discontinuation of Mass Water Fluoridation— It Can Be done!

1996: Water Authority of Western Nassau County, New York, voted 8 to 1 to discontinue their water fluoridation after 23 years.

1996: City of Worcester, Massachusetts, discontinued fluoridation.

1997: Yardley Borough, Bucks County, Pennsylvania. Fluoridation issue was defeated.

The piped water of Kuopio, Finland, was fluoridated in 1959 but stopped by strong opposition at the end of 1992. In 1995, a decrease in caries was seen in a nonfluoridated town that had been observed and in Kuopio. The study's conclusion was that the decrease in caries had little to do with whatever dentists were doing or with the water supply (L. Seppa, S. Karkkainen, H. Hausen. Caries frequency in permanent teeth before and after discontinuation of water fluoridation in Kuopio, Finland. Abstract from *Community Dentistry & Oral Epidemiology* 26 [4] 256-262 1998).

Researchers in Finland also found that people who lived 10 years or more in Kuopio, before fluoridation was stopped had extremely high levels of fluoride in their bones—thousands of parts per million—especially osteoporosis sufferers and people with impaired kidney function (E.M. Alhava, H. Olkkomen, P. Kauranen, T. Kari. The effect of drinking water fluoridation on the fluoride content, strength and mineral density of human bone, *Acta Orthopædica Scandinavica* 51 413-420 1980; I. Arnala, E.M., Alhava, E.M. Kauranen. Effects of fluoride on bone in Finland. Histomorphometry of cadaver bone from low and high fluoride areas, *Acta Orthopædica Scandinavica* 56 161-166 1985). After this research was published, Finland stopped fluoridation altogether.

One researcher thinks that a rise in the standard of living of many people may explain why tooth decay is declining. In New Zealand, for example, since the 1930s, there has been a tremendous increase in the consumption of fresh fruit and vegetables (V. Hamilton, J.A. Birkbeck. The Home Style Survey of New Zealand's Changing Diet. Quality Bakers, Palmerston North 1985) and an eightfold increase in the eating of cheese, which has anti-decay properties (E.L. Herod. The effect of cheese on dental caries: A review of the literature, *Australian Dental Journal* 36 (2)120-125 1991).

They Said It Themselves

Position of the American Dietetic Association (ADA):
The impact of fluoride on dental health
Journal of the American Dietetic Association 94(1994):1428–1431

"Once absorbed into the bloodstream, fluoride is either deposited into bones and developing teeth or excreted in the urine."

"Dietary fluoridation is contraindicated if the water is already optimally fluoridated, because dental fluorosis may result in children who consume excessive fluoride during the early stages of tooth development."

The American Dietetic Association notes that there has been an increase in the prevalence of mild fluorosis in recent years, which they attribute to the improper use of dietary fluoride supplements; ingestion of toothpastes and oral gels which should not be swallowed but sometimes are), and fluoride from foods and beverages processed in fluoridated areas and consumed by people in fluoridated as well as nonfluoridated areas.

According to the ADA, "Because foods processed with fluoridated water can add notably to total fluoride consumption (particularly in infants), potential sources of high fluoride intake in children's diets should be identified before any supplementation is recommended (N. G. Chaudhury, R. H. Brown, and M. G. Shepherd. "Fluoride Intake of Infants in New Zealand," *Journal of Dental Research* 69, 12 (1990): 828–1833).

APPENDIX C

Other Names for Thimerosal:

Mercurochrome®
Merthiolate®
Sodium ethylmercurithiosalicylate
Mercurothiolate
Merzonin
Mertorgan
Merfamin
Ethyl (2-mercaptobenzoato-S)mercury sodium salt
Thiomersalate
Thiomersal
Thiomersalan
[(o-carboxyphenyl)thio] ethylmercury sodium salt

Food Sources of Nutrients That Counteract Mercury

Nutrient	Food	Amount	Content (grams)
Cysteine	Granola	1 cup	0.30
	Oat flakes	1 cup	0.20
	Cheese	1 ounce	0.03
	Egg	one	0.07
	Whole milk	1 cup	0.07
	Yogurt	1 cup	0.93
Methionine	Granola	1 cup	0.20
	Oat flakes	1 cup	0.20
	Cheese	1 ounce	0.17
	Egg	one	0.20
	Whole milk	1 cup	0.20
	Yogurt	1 cup	0.23
Taurine	Fish and animal protein contain high concentrations of taurine.		
	It is not found in vegetable protein sources.		
	It is the second most abundant amino acid in human milk.		

SOURCE: E. R. Braverman, C. C. Pfeiffer, K. Blum, and R. Smayda, *The Healing Nutrients Within: Facts, Findings and New Research on Amino Acids*. (New Canaan, Conn: Keats Publishing, 1997).

Nutrient	Food	Amount	Content (milligrams)
Vitamin C	Orange	1 medium	70
	Apple + skin	1 medium	8
	Kiwi fruit	1 medium	74
	Broccoli	½ cup	37
	Carrots	½ cup	2
Vitamin E	Apple + skin	1 medium	1
	Mango	1 medium	2
	Broccoli	½ cup	1
	Carrots	½ cup	1
	Spinach	½ cup	2

SOURCE: Jean Barilla, *The Nutrition Superbook*, Volume 1: *The Antioxidants*. (New Canaan, Conn.: Keats Publishing, 1995).

Nutrient	Food	Content (milligrams) per 100 grams
Zinc	Peas	4.0
	Carrots	2.0
	Tomato	.24
	Oysters	143.0
	Beef liver	5.5
	Chicken breast	1.1
	Wheat bran	14.0
	Whole oatmeal	14.0
	Whole corn cereal	2.5
	Whole wheat bread	1.04
	White bread	0.12
	Peanut butter	2.0
	Whole egg	1.5
	Cow's milk	17–66

SOURCE: Carl C. Pfeiffer, *Mental and Elemental Nutrients*. (New Canaan, CT: Keats Publishing, 1975).

Nutrient	Food	Content (milligrams) per 100 grams
Magnesium	Almonds	270
	Peanuts	175
	Tofu	111
	Wheat grain	160
	Brown rice	88
	Milk	13
	Beef	21
	Chicken	19
	Banana	33
	Tomato	14
	Beets	25
	Buckwheat	229

Nutrient	Food	Content (milligrams) per 100 grams
Calcium	Cheddar cheese	750
	Collard leaves	250
	Almonds	234
	Figs, dried	126
	Yogurt	120
	Whole milk	118
	Cottage cheese	94
	Raisins	62
	Carrot	37
	Orange	31
	Tofu	128
	Beans, cooked, dry	50

Nutrient	Food	Amount	Grams of Fiber
Fiber	Apple + skin	1 medium	3.5
	Banana	1 medium	2.4
	Strawberries	1 cup	3.0
	Celery, raw	½ cup	1.1
	Green beans	1 cup	3.2

Fiber	Carrots	1 cup	4.6
(cont'd)	Potato + skin	1 medium	2.5
	Baked beans	½ cup	8.8
	Bread, whole wheat	1 slice	1.4
	Bread, white	1 slice	0.4
	Spaghetti	½ cup	1.1
	Oatmeal	¾ cup	1.6
	Shredded wheat	⅔ cup	2.6
	Almonds	10 nuts	1.1
	Peanuts	10 nuts	1.4

SOURCE: Michael T. Murray, *Encyclopedia of Nutritional Supplements* (Rocklin, Calif.: Prima Health, 1996).

Resources

Chapter 2

Information Services on Teratology and Reproductive Risk

Numerous teratogen information services are available throughout the United States. For information on the teratogen service in a particular area:

Eastern United States
Massachusetts Teratogen Information Service
Boston, Massachusetts
(617) 466-8474

Western United States
Pregnancy Riskline
Salt Lake City, Utah
(801) 328-2229

Computer Databases

Micromedex, Inc.
REPRORISK (REPROTEXT, REPROTOX, Shepard's Catalog of Teratogenic Agents, and TERIS) Englewood, CO

(800) 525-9083

National Library of Medicine, MEDLARS Service Dest
GRATEFUL MED (TOXLINE, TOXNET, and MEDLINE)
Bethesda, MD
(800) 638-8480

Reproductive Toxicology Center
REPROTOX
Columbia Hospital for Women Medical Center
Washington, DC
(202) 293-5137

Shepard's Catalog of Teratogenic Agents
University of Washington
Seattle, WA
(206) 543-3373

Teratogen Information System
TERIS and Shepard's Catalog of Teratogenic Agents
Seattle, WA
(206) 543-2465

Chapter 3

La Leche League International
P.O. Box 4079
Schaumburg, IL 60168-4079
(847) 519-9585

Food and Drug Administration (FDA)
To report an adverse event or illness believed to be related to the
use of an infant formula:
(800) FDA-1088 or website: *www.fda.gov/medwatch/report/con-
sumer/consumer.htm*

Chapter 4

For information on myofunctional therapy (tongue-thrust correction) contact:

International Association of Orofacial Myology
Jeanne Spahn, MA
970 South Elizabeth St.
Denver, CO 80209
Telephone (303) 765-4395
FAX (303) 733-8006
for the organization e-mail: *iaomoffice@aol/com*
Website: *www.iaom.com*
    (This group has a number of members in the U.S. and Canada, and in other countries, too, who do myofunctional therapy).

American Myofunctional Therapy Center
27 Mirror Lake Estates Drive
Whitefield, NH 03598
(603) 837-3400
    (This is the office of Susie Swenson, Garliner-trained and active in the IAOM. She will also give referrals to myofunctional therapists).

American Speech and Hearing Association
(800) 498-2071
    Ask for the Action Center for referral to a speech therapist who does myofunctional therapy—they may call it "tongue-thrust correction."

Barbara Greene, MFT
222 Meigs Road #12
Santa Barbara, CA 93109-1964
(805) 964-5903 *www.tonguethrust.com*
    (She is a Garliner-trained therapist who will give referrals to myofunctional therapists and has a very informative web site.)

Nuk Orthodontic Exerciser/Pacifier by Gerber
Gerber Products Company
c/o Consumer Affairs
445 State Street
Fremont, MI 49413-0001
For immediate answers any time day or night,
call (800) 4-GERBER.
www.gerber.com

My Thumb and I, Carol Mayer, M.S.
(800) 337-9049
www.thumbco.com

Mr. Wizard's Thumbs Out, Linda Bejoian, M.S.
(800) 829-4435

Chapter 5

Laclede, Inc.
Rancho Dominguez, CA 90220
(800) 922-5856

Rota-dent made by
Pro-Dentec
Batesville, AK 72503
http://www.prodentec.com

POH
Oral Health Products, Inc.
P.O. Box 470623
Tulsa, OK 74147
(800) 331-4645
www.oralhealthproducts.com

Chapter 6

The Natural Dentist
Fort Lee, NJ
(800) 827-5617

Chapter 10

Resource: New York State Coalition Opposed to Fluoridation, Inc.
P.O. Box 263, Old Bethpage, NY 11804
Carol Kopf (516) 796-5336, Evelyn Hannan (516) 378-7309

Citizens for Safe Drinking Water, (800) 728-3833

The Holistic Dental Association, e-mail: *hda@frontier.net, website:
www.holisticdental,org*
P. O. Box 5007
Durango, CO 81301

The Safe Water Foundation
6439 Taggart Road
Delaware, OH 43015

Agency for Toxic Substances and Disease Registry
Division of Toxicology
1600 Clifton Road NE, Mailstop E-29
Atlanta, GA 30333
Phone (800) 447-1544
FAX: (404) 639-6315

Chapter 12

John O. Butler Company (for orthodontic toothbrushes)
(800) JBUTLER
www.jbutler.com

General Resources

American Academy of Pediatric Dentistry. (AAPD)
http://www.aapd.org
211 East Chicago Avenue
Chicago, IL 60611-2663
(312) 377-2169
FAX (312) 337-6329

American Dental Association (ADA) *www.ada.org*
211 E. Chicago Ave.
Chicago, IL 60611
(312) 440-2500
FAX (312) 440-2800

Organizations

Price-Pottenger Nutrition Foundation. PO Box 2614, LaMesa CA, 91943-2614. (800) 366-3748. Membership includes a subscription to their quarterly Journal, plus other membership benefits. They carry a number of the books we have listed.

Holistic Dental Association. Richard Shepard, DDS, Exec. Director, PO Box 5007, Durango, CO. 81301, (970) 259-1091 *www.holisticdental.org.* This organization has many dentist members across the US.

International Academy of Oral Medicine and Toxicology. PO Box 608531, Orlando, FL, 32860-8531, (407) 298-2450, (407) 298-3075 (FAX). Dentists who are members have knowledge and expertise in removing mercury fillings, and in other holistic approaches.

La Leche League, 1400 N. Meacham Rd., Schaumburg, IL, 60173-4048. *www.lalecheleague.org.* Provides education, information, and support through local chapters across the country, for women who want to breast feed.

International Association of Orofacial Myology, 970 Elizabeth Street, Denver, CO 80209. *www.iaom.com.* This group has members in the US and Canada who do myofunctional therapy and work with thumb-sucking problems.

American Speech and Hearing Association. Call (800) 498-2071 and ask for the Action Center for a referral to a speech therapist in your area who does myofunctional therapy (also called tongue thrust therapy).

American Society for the Study of Orthodontics. Contact: Exec. Director Ms. Daisy Buchalter, 50-12 204th St., Flushing, NY 11364 (718) 224-8898 for a referral to a dentist member who does removable appliance orthodontic treatment.

Safe Water Foundation 6439 Taggart Rd., Delaware, OH 43015. Information on fluoride and other toxins in your water.

Bibliography

BOOKS

Brewer, Gail Sforza with Thomas H. Brewer, M.D., medical consultant. *The Brewer Medical Diet for Normal and High-Risk Pregnancy.* New York: Simon and Schuster (Fireside), 1983. A leading obstetrician's guide to every stage of pregnancy.

Brewer, Thomas H. *Metabolic Toxemia of Late Pregnancy.* New Canaan, CT: Keats Publishing, 1982

Chancellor, Philip M. *Dr. Philip M. Chancellor's Handbook of the Bach Flower Remedies,* New Canaan, CT: Keats Publishing, Inc., 1971, 1980. Contains information on prescribing the Remedies for children.

Cheraksin, Emanuel, M.D., D.M.D., W. Marshall Ringsdorf, Jr., D.M.D., and James W. Clark, D.D.S. *Diet and Disease.* New Canaan, CT: Keats Publishing 1968, 1995. The classic work on the relationship between health and nutrition.

Crook, William G., M.D. *Help for the Hyperactive Child.* Jackson, TN: Professional Books, 1991. Important information on how diet can cause many childhood illnesses as well as behavior problems. By the author of *The Yeast Connection.*

Dufty, William. *Sugar Blues.* Radnor PA: Chilton Book Co., 1975. The politics and perils of sugar.

Fallon, Sally. *Nourishing Traditions.* Washington, D.C.: New Trends Publishing, 1999. A cookbook and a guide to wise food choices and proper food preparation techniques for optimum nutrition.

Goldbeck, Nikki. *As You Eat So Your Baby Grows: A Guide to Nutrition in Pregnancy.* Woodstock, NY: Ceres Press, 2000. A concise booklet with important information. From: PO Box 87, Woodstock, NY 12498. Phone/FAX (914) 679-5573.

Kennedy, David, D.D.S. *How to Save Your Teeth: Toxic-Free Preventive Dentistry.* Delaware, OH: Health Action Press, 1993. Good advice from a holistic dentist.

Mayer, Carol A., M.S., C.C.C./S.P. & C.O.M. *My Thumb and I.* Temecula, CA: Speech Dynamics, Inc. 2000. How to stop a finger or thumb-sucking habit, guidelines for parents and fun activities for the child.

Meinig, George, D.D.S. *"NEW" trition.* Ojai, CA: Bion Publishing, 1987. Excellent nutrition advice in a question and answer format.

Mendelsohn, Robert S., M.D. *How to Raise a Healthy Child In Spite of Your Doctor.* New York: Ballantine Books, 1984. What parents need to know when making health decisions for their children.

Montagu, Ashley, Ph. D. *Prenatal Influences.* Springfield, IL: Charles C. Thomas, 1961.

Moore, Keith L., ed. *The Developing Human.* 3rd Edition, Philadelphia, PA: W.B. Saunders Company, 1982.

Murray, Michael and Pizzorno, Joseph. *Encyclopedia of Natural Medicine.* Revised 2nd Ed. Rocklin, CA: Prima Publishing, 1998. A good information source.

Panos, Maesimund, B., M.D. and Jane Heimlich. *Homeopathic Medicine at Home: Natural Remedies for Everyday Ailments and Minor Injuries.* Los Angeles, CA: J.P. Tarcher, 1980. This easy-to-use guide to homeopathic remedies is one of the best.

Pennybacker, Mindy. *Non-Toxic and Friendly Way to Take Care of Your Child.* New York: John Wiley & Sons, 1999. Good advice on children's health.

Pescatore, Fred, M.D. *Feed Your Kids Well: How to Help Your Child Lose Weight and Get Healthy.* New York: John Wiley & Sons, 1998. This is not just for children who need to lose weight, it has advice for coping with childhood illnesses and helping children to optimal health.

Price, Weston, DDS. *Nutrition and Physical Degeneration.* New Caan, CT: Keats Publishing, 1939 (Reprinted 1989). This classic study of peoples in all parts of the world who had remarkable health while eating their native diets, but suffered devastating reverses in health after starting to eat processed "modern" food.

Rasmussen, Bettina B. Danish Holistic Clinic. *Bach Flower Essences & Children.* Accessed 10/30/00 at: *www.organix.net/organix/bachc.htm*

Weiss, Jay, D.M.D. *Embraceable You: A Guide for Orthodontic Patients and their Parents.* New York: Health Sciences Publishing, 1975.

Williams, Roger J., Ph.D. *Biochemical Individuality.* New Canaan, CT: Keats Publishing, 1956, (Reprinted 1998). This is a classic book on nutrition. It tells how nutrition is linked to our genetic differences.

Yiamouyiannis, John, Ph. D. *Fluoride: The Aging Factor.* Delaware,

OH: Health Action Press, 1983. This is the classic book on fluoride toxicity, the lack of efficacy of fluoride in preventing cavities, and the many health problems it causes.

Ziff, Sam, Ph. D. *Silver Dental Fillings: The Toxic Time Bomb.* New York: Aurora Press, 1984. An in-depth perspective on the hazards of mercury from silver fillings.

Ziff, Sam, and Michael Ziff. *Infertility & Birth Defects: Is mercury from silver dental fillings an unsuspected cause?* Orlando, FL: Bio-Probe, 1987.

Video Cassettes

Mr. Wizard's Thumb's Out by Linda BeJoian, M.S., speech pathologist and myofunctional therapist. Motivates children with an excellent program for overcoming the thumb habit. Call (800) 829-4435.

Taming the Tongue Thrust by Suzanne Barnes, M.A. An effective program for retraining the tongue for children who have a tongue thrust or incorrect swallow; a program of guided myofunctional therapy. Call (626) 355-1729. Address: 55 N. Auburn, Suite A, Sierra Madre, CA 91024. Website: *www.suzspeech.com* ; e-mail: *SuzSpeech@aol.com* .

Magazines

Better Nutrition, Sabot Publishing. Free at your local health store or call: (203) 321-1722. The latest nutrition news.

Mothering. P.O. Box 1690, Santa Fe, NM 87504-9774. Call (800) 984-8116 A holistic and humanistic viewpoint and lots of helpful information for raising healthy children.

Townsend Letter for Doctors and Patients. Edited by Jonathan Collin, MD. 911 Tyler St., Pt. Townsend, WA 98368-6541. Call

(360) 385-6021; (360) 385-0699 (FAX). Website: *www.tldp.com*. The latest information on holistic health written by researchers, health practitioners, and patients.

Vegetarian Times, 4 High Ridge Park, Stamford, CT 06907 (203) 328-7040; FAX (203) 328-7078. On the web: *www.vegetariantimes.com*. For vegetarian recipes.

Newsletters

Bio-Probe Newsletter. 5508 Edgewater Dr., Orlando FL. 32810. Call (407) 290-9670. $75 per year, bimonthly. Website: *www.bioprobe.com* . Information on toxic substances such as mercury used in dental procedures.

The Holistic Dental Digest—PLUS edited by Jerry Mittelman, D.D.S. and Beverly Mittelman B.S., 263 West End Ave., #2A, New York, NY 10023. $13.25 per year, bimonthly. E-mail: *hdd@bway.net* Succinct information you're not likely to get elsewhere on dental and health subjects, plus a referral list of dentists, physicians, and myofunctional therapists. Call (212) 874-4212.

SUPPLEMENTS, FOODS, AND OTHER PRODUCTS

The following companies have a number of products listed in this resource section. Companies with only one product listed have their toll-free numbers and web sites listed along with their products.

Carlson® Laboratories
888-234-5656
www.carlsonlabs.com

Carotec, Inc.
800-522-4279
www.carotec.com

Jarrow Formulas™
800-726-0886
www.jarrow.com

MegaFood™
800-848-2542
www.megafood.com

Moss Nutrition
800-851-5444
www.mossnutrition.com
A resource for doctors
and dentists to use. It
offers specialty supplements
that can be ordered only by
your physician or dentist.

N.E.E.D.S.
800-634-1380
www.needs.com
This is a mail order company offering a full line of quality supplements from top companies including Solgar, Source Naturals®, Carlson, Tyler, Nature's Way, and Nutricology.

Omega Nutrition
800-661-3529
www.omeganutrition.com

Source Naturals®
800-815-2333
www.sourcenaturals.com

Tishcon Corporation
800-848-8442
www.tishcon.com
Raw goods supplier.

Tree of Life®
www.treeoflife.com

Supplements

Prenatal Formulas

Carlson®
Pre-natal
A multiple vitamin-and-mineral supplement formulated for the special needs of pregnant and lactating women. Vegetarian, natural-source vitamins and minerals, natural color and sugar free. Tablet form.

MegaFood™
Baby & Me DailyFoods®
A carefully balanced vitamin, mineral, and herbal formula with 100% complex FoodState® nutrients, which are gentle on the stomach. Nutritional support to meet the special challenges of pregnancy and lactation. Recommendation is six tablets daily, which can be taken even on an empty stomach or sprinkled on food.

Moss Nutrition
preMA™ Prenatal Powder
A prenatal vitamin-and-mineral product in a powdered drink mix form. Contains 1,000 mg of calcium and 500 mg of magnesium per serving. Preferred by patients who would rather not swallow pills. Preservative and excipient free. One level scoop provides vitamins A, C, D, E, thiamin, riboflavin, niacin, B-6, folate, B-12, biotin, and panthothenic acid, and the minerals iodine, magnesium, zinc, selenium, copper, manganese, chromium, and molybdenum.

N.E.E.D.S.
Prenatal Capsule
Complete professional multi-vitamin-and-mineral formula.
Supplied by Tyler.

Children's Formulas

Multiple Vitamins and Minerals

Carlson®
Scooter Rabbit
A multiple vitamin-and-mineral product containing vitamins A, C, D, E, K, B-1, B-2, niacin, biotin, B-6, folate, B-12, biotin and pantothenic acid, and all the important minerals. Includes sweeteners naturally found in fruit, such as sorbitol and fructose.

MegaFood™
Kids & Us™, Mini's™
A Full Color Spectrum FoodBased Nutrition™ containing vitamins, minerals, and tonic herbs in pea-size easy-to-swallow tablets. Listed as 72% whole food.

Moss Nutrition
Aqueous Multi-Plus™
A liquid multiple vitamin-and-mineral product designed for children but also used by adults who have problems swallowing capsules or tablets. Contains vitamins A, C, D, E, K, B-1, B-2, niacin, biotin, B-6, B-12, and pantothenic acid, and all the important minerals.

N.E.E.D.S.
Children's Multiple Drop
One dropperful (20 drops) per day can be added to juice or water. A complete vitamin-and-mineral formulation. No sugar added. For children ages 1 through 4. Supplied by Metagenics.

Children's Multi-Vitamin Capsule
No sugar added. Can be opened and sprinkled onto food. One capsule for each 10 lbs. of body weight. No sugar added. Supplied by Nutricology.

Source Naturals®
Mega-Kid™Multiple
A complete, high-potency, pleasant-tasting, chewable vitamin, designed to meet the nutritional needs of growing children. Two tablets contain vitamins A, B-1, B-2, niacinamide, B-5, B-6, B-12, biotin, folic acid, C, D-3, E, and K, and all the important minerals. Also include bioflavonoids, bee pollen, and digestive enzymes (papaya). For children ages 1 through 3, one tablet daily; ages 4 through 6, two tablets daily; ages 7 through 10, three tablets daily.

Vitamin A

Moss Nutrition
Bio-AE-Mulsion
An emulsified form of vitamin A. Because the emulsification process creates such a small particle size, the vitamin A in the product requires little or no liver metabolism. This, plus the fact that Bio-AE-Mulsion is provided in a liquid form, makes it ideal for use with children. Each drop supplies 2,000 IU. Also for adults.

Vitamin C

Carlson®
Scooter Rabbit-C
Chewable vitamin C tablets that contain 250 mg of vitamin C and 25 mg of calcium as calcium ascorbate, which is gentle on the stomach.

Vitamin D

Moss Nutrition
Bio-D-Mulsion
An oil-in-water emulsion in which vitamin D has been dispersed. Each drop supplies 400 IU of emulsified vitamin D.

Special Children's Formulas

Source Naturals®
Focus Child™
Designed to support your child's ability to focus. Each ingredient has its own unique and powerful action. DMAE, a substance normally found in the brain, has been shown to help enhance mental concentration. DHA is a fatty acid the brain uses for its growth and function. Studies have shown that very active children may have special dietary needs for DHA, magnesium, and zinc. Magnesium plays a role in neuromuscular transmission and activity. L-aspartate, an amino acid, acts as a neurotransmitter. Grape seed extract is rich in proanthocyanidins, which have powerful antioxidant activity. Phosphatidylserine is a vital component of cell membranes, including those in the brain. Two tablets contain magnesium, zinc, L-aspartate, DMAE, standardized soybean lecithin, (LECI-PS®) (20 mg phosphatidylserine, 6 mg phosphatidylcholine, 3.5 mg phosphatidylethanolamine, 1 mg phosphatidylinositol), 15 mg DHA (Neuromins™), and 15 mg grape seed extract.

Adult Formulas

Amino Acids

Before birth, the enzymes necessary to get cysteine into the brain are not present. So the unborn baby depends on the mother's blood as a source of cysteine. Taurine is made from cysteine, so it's imortant that the mother have a good supply. This sulfur-containing amino acid is highly concentrated in the brain, where it can protect the brain cells and help them function properly. The amounts of taurine are high in the fetal liver and brain, and some researchers think that taurine helps brain development.

Carlson®
The following amino acids are available as a free-form powder in bottles of 100 grams:
L-cysteine, L-methionine, and L-taurine. Serving size is 1 tsp.

Source Naturals®
L-cysteine
Mono HCL powder.
¼ tsp. contains approximately 627 mg of L-cysteine.

L-methionine
Free form powder
¼ tsp. contains approximately 627 mg of L-methionine.

Taurine
Free form powder
¼ tsp. contains approximately 675 mg of L-taurine.

Antioxidants

MegaFood™
Antioxidant DailyFoods® Vitamin, Mineral & Herbal Formula
Contains vitamins A, C, and E, zinc, and selenium. DailyFoods® FoodState® nutrients are 100% Whole Food and can be taken at any time of the day, even on an empty stomach. Tablet form.

Tishcon Corporation
Super Antioxidant Supreme
Two softgels contain 200 IU of vitamin E, (d-alpha-tocopherol plus mixed tocopherols), B-6, B-12, folic acid, selenium, alpha lipoic acid, lutein, lycopene, L-glutathione, and other powerful nutrients.

Tishcon's Super Antioxidant Supreme is available from the following companies:

Phytotherapy: 201-891-1104
Epic: 800-866-0978
Optimum Health: 800-228-1507
Doctor's Preferred: 800-304-1708
Solanova: 800-200-0456

Beta-Carotene

Carlson®
Caro Plete®
Alpha- and beta-carotene and other carotenoids.

Super Beta-Carotene
16 mg of natural D. salina (plant algae) provides 25,000 IU of vitamin A activity. No synthetic solvents, preservatives, or additives are used. Softgel form.

Carotec
Carotenoids
Each softgel contains 6 mg lutein, 7.5 mg lycopene, 256 mcg zeaxanthin, 6.8 mg beta-carotene, and 3.6 mg alpha-carotene

N.E.E.D.S.
Beta Carotene
Each softgel contains 25,000 IU.
Supplied by Nature's Way.

Source Naturals®
Beta-Carotene
Each softgel contains vitamin A activity 25,000 IU (from 15 mg of beta-carotene).

Super Beta-Carotene
Natural D salina derived from the sea plant Dunaliella salina. Each softgel also contains vitamin A.

Calcium

Carlson®
Chelated Cal-Mag
Two tablets contain 400 mg calcium and 200 mg magnesium from 333 mg of calcium and magnesium chelates.

Liquid Cal-Mag
Two softgels contain 400 mg calcium and 200 mg magnesium with vitamin D.

N.E.E.D.S.
Calcium/Magnesium
Two tablets contain 1000 mg of calcium and 500 mg of magnesium.
Supplied by Company Now.

Omega Nutrition
Liquid Life Essential Night Formula
A mineral-rich formula with a pleasant coconut flavor that is designed to help tissue repair and calcium assimilation while you sleep. Suitable for all members of the family. Supplied by Holistic Enterprises.

Source Naturals®
Calcium-Magnesium, Amino Acid Chelate
Calcium and magnesium work together in several key physiological processes. They are important in the regulation of blood pressure and for healthy muscle function. Both are components of skeletal tissue, and magnesium is necessary for calcium's absorption into the bones. Each tablet contains 250 mg calcium, 125 mg magnesium, and 500 IU vitamin D.

Coenzyme Q10

Carlson®
Co-Q10
Available in 10 mg, 30 mg, 50 mg, 100 mg, and 200 mg softgels.

Carotec
CocoQ-10® 100
Each softgel contains 100 mg coenzyme Q-10 and 250 mg coconut oil.

Source Naturals®
Coenzyme Q10
Available in 30 mg and 100 mg softgels.

Tishcon Corporation
Hydrosoluble CoQ10 with high bioavailability. Available in softsules® (softgels) in the following doses:
Q-Gel®, 15 mg
Q-Gel® Forte, 30 mg
Q-Gel® Plus, 30 mg CoQ10, 50 mg alpha lipoic acid, and 100 IU natural vitamin E
Q-Gel® Ultra: 60 mg

Carni-Q-Gel®, 30 mg CoQ10 and 250 mg L-carnitine

Tishcon's CoQ10 products are available from the following companies:

Bio Energy Nutrients (a division of Whole Foods): 800-627-7775
Physiologics (a division of Whole Foods): 800-765-6775
CountryLife: 631-231-1031
Solanova: 800-200-0456
Phytotherapy: 201-891-1104
Nutrimedika: 800-688-7462
Swanson: 800-437-4148
Jordets: 888-816-7676
Epic: 800-866-0978
Optimum Health: 800-228-1507
Doctor's Preferred: 800-304-1708

Omega-3 Essential Fatty Acids

Taking Omega-3 oils in supplement form is recommended for many conditions. This is because omega-3 is part of the essential fatty acids that are necessary for health. It is found in fish oils—such as cod liver and salmon—and flaxseed oil, as well as in a non-fish, micro-algae form (Neuromins® DHA).

DHA

DHA, an essential fatty acid necessary for life, is available in a non-fish, micro-algae form (for those who don't want to use fish products). Look for a product called Neuromins® DHA (in softgel form). Because of the importance of this product, several leading supplement companies are marketing Neuromins® DHA to health food and other stores. Listed below are companies, along with their customer service numbers, that can direct you to where to obtain this product in your area:

BioDynamax (AMRION):	800-926-7525
Carotec:	800-522-4279
Moss Nutrition:	800-851-5444
Natrol®:	800-326-1520
Nature's Way:	800-962-8873
Solaray (Nutraceutical Corp.):	800-683-9640
Solgar:	800-645-2246
Source Naturals:	800-815-2333
Your Life (Leiner):	800-533-8482

Neuromins® DHA is available at health-food stores everywhere, including the following:

Vitamin Shoppe:	800-223-1216
Vitamin World:	800-645-1030
Whole Food Markets:	800-901-0094
Wild Oats:	800-494-WILD

Mail-order sources for Neuromins® DHA:

Vitamin Shoppe:	800-223-1216
Puritan's Pride:	800-645-1030

On-line sources for Neuromins® DHA (use the search word "Neuromins" or "DHA"):

www.vitaminshoppe.com
www.mothernature.com
www.drugstore.com
www.puritan.com

Fish Oils

Carlson®
Norwegian Salmon Oil
Each softgel contains 1,000 mg of salmon oil. Two softgels contain 350 mg of total omega-3 fatty acids, including EPA (eicosapentaenoic acid), DHA (docosahexaenoic acid), DPA (docosapentaenoic acid) and ALA (alpha-liolenic acid).

Super-DHA™
Each softgel contains 1,000 mg of a special blend of fish body oils, including menhaden and sardines, which are high in DHA (docosahexaenoic acid) and EPA (eicosapentaenoic acid). This product is unique because it supplies 500 mg of DHA and 200 mg of EPA.

Super Omega-3 Fish Oils
Contains a special concentrate of fish body oils from deep, cold-water fish, including mackerel and sardines, which are especially rich in EPA and DHA. Each softgel contains 500 to 550 mg of total omega-3 fatty acids including 300 mg of EPA (eicosapentaenoic acid), and 200 mg of DHA (docosahexaenoic acid), and ALA (alpha-liolenic acid).

Source Naturals®
OmegaEPA™
Marine lipids with EPA and DHA
Each 1,000 mg softgel contains 180 mg of EPA and 120 mg of DHA.

OmegaFlax™
Fresh, Cold-Pressed Flaxseed Oil
Flaxseed oil is an ideal vegetarian source of omega-3 essential fatty acids. Each softgel contains 1,000 mg.

Flaxseed

Omega Nutrition
Hi-Lignan Nutri-Flax Capsules
Each capsule contains 550 mg powder. A high-lignan fiber product with 7.9 mg of lignans per three-capsule (1,650 mg) serving. Lignans are the metabolism-balancing phytochemicals in flax. Flax seed fiber contains 30% more lignans than whole flax seed.

Folic Acid

N.E.E.D.S.
Each capsule contains 800 mcg. Supplied by Nutrisupplies.

Garlic

Carlson®
Garlic-600
Orderless, high potency, coated tablets. Each tablet contains 600 mg.

Source Naturals®
Garlic Oil
Odorless and tasteless. Each softgel contains garlic oil extracted from 500 mg of fresh garlic bulb, in a base of soybean oil.

Wakunaga of America
800-421-2998
www.kyolic.com
Kyolic® Aged Garlic Extract (AGE)
The most scientifically researched garlic product in the world (over 220 studies). Available in capsules as well as liquid form (which can be added to food).

Ginger

Jarrow Formulas™
Freeze-Dried Ginger
Each capsule contains 500 mg of freeze dried ginger.

Garlic plus Ginger
Each capsule contains 500 mg of Jarro-Gar™ odor modified garlic and 200 mg of freeze-dried ginger (6:1 extract).

For a wonderful and extremely healthful ginger drink, see the "Tea" section under "Foods for Health."

Homeopathic Remedies

Liddell Laboratories
800-460-7733
www.liddell.net
A highly effective and easy to use homeopathic line of sublingual oral sprays. These products relieve a wide range of symptoms associated with such conditions as cold and flu, sinus congestion, allergy and hay fever, back pain, sciatica, arthritis, and stress. Formulated by a physician, all of Liddell's 130 spray products contain safe and effective natural ingredients. The new oral sprays allow exceptional absorption by the body and have been shown to work well in combination with other products such as dietary supplements and over-the-counter or prescription drugs.

Magnesium

Carlson®
Liquid Magnesium
Each softgel supplies 400 mg of magnesium from magnesium oxide.

Magnesium Capsules
Each capsule supplies 350 mg of magnesium from magnesium oxide.

Carotec
Tropocor
A magnesium aspartate and potassium aspartate combination. Each tablet contains 125 mg each of magnesium aspartate and potassium aspartate (8.3 mg elemental magnesium and 27.3 mg elemental potassium). Made to pharmaceutical standards.

Source Naturals®
Magnesium
Amino Acid Chelate
Each tablet contains 100 mg of magnesium (from 500 mg of magnesium amino acid chelate).

Vitamins

Vitamin A

Moss Nutrition
Bio-AE-Mulsion
An emulsified form of vitamin A. Because the emulsification process creates such a small particle size, the vitamin A in the product requires little or no liver metabolism. This, plus the fact that Bio-AE-Mulsion is provided in a liquid form, makes it ideal for use with children. Each drop supplies 2,000 IU.

N.E.E.D.S.
Vitamin A
Each softgel contains 10,000 I.U. Supplied by Nature's Way.

Vitamin B-6

Source Naturals®
Available in 50 mg, 100 mg, and 500 mg timed-release tablets.

Vitamin B-12

Carlson®
B-12 SL
Sublingual tablets that taste great.

N.E.E.D.S.
B-12
Each tablet contains 1,000 mcg. Supplied by Solgar.

Source Naturals®
Vitamin B-12, Vegetarian Sublingual
Each sublingual tablet contains 2,000 mcg. Sweetened wtih sorbitol and mannitol, and flavored with natural lemon.

Vitamin B Complex

Carlson®
B-Compleet™
Vitamin B Complex with 500 mg vitamin C. Provides all the B vitamins plus vitamin C in a balanced formulation. B-Compleet was formulated to meet the increased needs the body has for the water-soluble vitamins during stress.

Carotec
Bio B-Complex
Each capsule contains 25 mg of each of the "macro" B vitamins (B-1, B-2, B-3, B-6) and pantothenic acid, 25 mcg of B-12 and D-biotin, 200 mcg of folic acid, 80 mg of choline, 50 mg of inositol, 2 mg of PABA, plus 5 mg of Bioperine®, an ingredient that makes the B vitamins and other nutrients better absorbed and metabolized.

Source Naturals®
Coenzymate™ B Complex
Each sublingual tablet contains coenzymes along with a full range of B vitamins and CoQ10. Orange or peppermint flavored.

Vitamin C

Carlson®
Mild-C Chewable
Buffered form of chewable vitamin C that is non-acidic and gentle to the teeth. Each tablet contains 250 mg of vitamin C and 28 mg of calcium. Orange or tangerine flavored.

Carotec
Vitamin C Plus
Each capsule contains 500 mg of vitamin C as L-ascorbic acid, 50 mg of Leucoselect™ grape seed extract, 50 mg of hawthorne extract, and 100 mg of grape skin extract (contains resveratrol).

MegaFood™
Complex C
Vitamin C as found in food is a very complex nutrient of which ascorbic acid is only one factor. Complex C DailyFoods® contains all the food factors, such as bioflavonoids, that occur in food and enhance its effectiveness. DailyFoods® FoodState® nutrients are 100% Whole Food and can be taken at any time throughout the day, even on an empty stomach. Available in 250 mg tablets.

N.E.E.D.S.
Buffered Non-Corn Source Vitamin C
Each capsule contains 500 mg. Supplied by Nutricology.

Source Naturals®
C-500
Each tablet contains 500 mg of vitamin C (ascorbic acid) and 50 mg of rose hips.

Calcium Ascorbate, Vitamin C Crystals
Dissolve instantly. Each ¼ tsp. supplies 1,000 mg of vitamin C and 125 mg of calcium.

Magnesium Ascorbate
Crystals that dissolve instantly. Magnesium ascorbate is the nonacidic, buffered form of vitamin C. It is gentle on the stomach and provides an excellent source of the essential mineral magnesium. Each ¼ tsp. supplies 1,000 mg of vitamin C and 78 mg of magnesium.

Vitamin D

Carlson®
Vitamin D
Natural source of vitamin D_3 from fish liver oil. Available in 400 IU and 1,000 IU softgels.

Moss Nutrition
Bio-D-Mulsion
An oil-in-water emulsion in which vitamin D has been dispersed. Each drop supplies 400 IU of emulsified vitamin D.

N.E.E.D.S.
Vitamin D
Each tablet contains 400 I.U. Supplied by Vitaline.

Source Naturals®
Vitamin A and D
Each tablet contains 10,000 IU of vitamin A (palmitate) and 400 IU of vitamin D (cholecalciferol). Vitamin D is an essential nutrient that helps regulate calcium and phosphorous levels in the bones, teeth, and blood. It is necessary for the proper absorption of calcium from the intestines and for the normal mineralization of bones.

Vitamin E

Carlson®
E-Gems® Elite
E-Gems Elite is an exclusive All-Natural Vitamin E formula providing the complete E-Family of Tocopherols & Tocotrienols (very important antiodidants). Each easy-to-swallow softgel provides 400 IU of Vitamin E plus 100 mg. of d-Gamma Tocopherol, 40 mg. of d-Beta and d-Delta Tocopherol, and 20 mg. of d-Gamma, d-Alpha, d-Beta and d-Delta Tocotrienols.

Carlson®
d-Alpha Gems™
Each softgel contains 400 IU of vitamin E (d-alpha tocopherol acetate).

E-Gems® Plus
All natural vitamin E derived from soybean oil, supplying alpha-tocopherol plus mixed tocopherols. Available in 200 IU, 400 IU, and 800 IU softgels.

Carotec
"The" Vitamin E
Each softgel contains 200 IU of alpha tocopherol, 75 mg of gamma tocopherol, 28 mg of delta tocopherol, and 1 mg of beta tocopherol.

MegaFood™
E and Selenium DailyFoods®
In foods, vitamin E and selenium are always found together, since they need each other to work. This combination offers these two important nutrients as they naturally occur in food and therefore provides maximum protection. DAILY-FOODS® FoodState® nutrients are 100% Whole Food and can be taken at any time throughout the day, even on an empty stomach. Each tablet contains 100 IU of vitamin E and 100 mg of selenium.

Source Naturals®
Vitamin E
Each softgel contains 400 IU of natural vitamin E (d-alpha tocopherol) and 67 mg of mixed tocopherols (d-beta, d-gamma, and d-delta). In a base of soybean oil.

Tocotrienols

Carotec
Palm Tocotrienols
Each softgel contains 200 mg palm derived tocotrienols.

Source Naturals®
Tocotrienol Antioxidant Complex™
Each softgel contains a total of 34 mg of tocotrienols (29.8 of gamma-tocotrienol, 3 mg of alpha-tocotrienol, and 1.3 mg of delta-tocotrienol) and 100 IU of vitamin E (d-alpha tocopherol).

Multivitamin and Multimineral Formulations

Carlson® Laboratories
Super-1-Daily
A super-strength multi-vitamin and -mineral formula. Vegetarian; free of animal, fish, and dairy. Tablet form.

MegaFood™
LIFESTYLE™ DAILYFOODS® Vitamin, Mineral and Herbal Formula
This unique formulation delivers nutrients in the FoodState® for maximum utilization. Recent scientific studies have proven that nutrients function at their peak when consumed as they naturally occur in food. Because MegaFood™'s formulas are food, they are particularly effective. DailyFoods® FoodState® nutrients are 100% Whole Food and can be taken at any time throughout the day, even on an empty stomach. Tablet form.

Women's DailyFoods®
A vitamin, mineral, and herbal formula for women in all the cycles of life. Daily-
Foods® FoodState® nutrients are 100% Whole Food and can be taken at any time
throughout the day, even on an empty stomach. Three tablets daily.

Source Naturals®
Élan Vitàl™ Multiple
Significant potencies of standard nutrients. Provides antioxidant protection, aids
cellular energy metabolism and neurotransmitter production, and supports the
liver, the key organ of nutrient activity. Six tablets contain a full supply of all necessary vitamins and minerals.

Zinc

Carlson®
Zinc
Contains zinc from zinc gluconate. Available in 15 mg and 50 mg tablets.

Carotec
Unizink
50 mg zinc aspartate (9.9 mg elemental zinc). Made to pharmaceutical standards.

N.E.E.D.S.
Zinc Picolinate
Each capsule contains 30 mg. Supplied by Nutrisupplies.

Source Naturals®
OptiZinc®
Each tablet contains 30 mg of zinc from 150 mg of OptiZinc® zinc monomethio-
nine.

Foods for Health

Cheeses

Country Hills Organic, Inc.
330-893-2596

Pure Pastures Organic Cheese
A complete family of delicious and healthy organic cheeses that are produced in
accordance with the 1990 California Organic Foods Act. Country Hills' dairy
farmers are overseen by the Ohio Ecological Food and Farm Association (OEFFA)
and raise their cattle on organic grains and feed. Herds are free of chemicals, artificial growth hormones, and antibiotics. All of their products are made with 100%
certified organic milk and ingredients that are certified organic by Quality
Assurance International (QAI). Their cheeses are available in six traditional styles,
including Cheddar, Colby, Swiss, and Havarti, as well as in an assortment of yogurt cheeses.

Tree of Life
Organic Cheeses, including Colby, Cheddar, Jalapeño Jack, Mozarella, Provolone, and Swiss. These wonderful cheeses are available at many health food stores.

Fish Oils

Carlson®
Norwegian Cod Liver Oil
Liquid form. High in omega-3 and other essential fatty acids and vitamin E. Natural and lemon flavored. Can be mixed into food. For all members of the family, especially children.

Grains

INF-InterNatural Foods
201-909-0808

McCann's Steelcut Wholegrain Irish Oatmeal
High in B vitamins, calcium, protein, and fiber, while low in fat with no added salt.

Lundberg Family Farms
530-882-4550 (ext. 319)
www.lundberg.com

A full line of organic and exotic rice.

Meats

D'Artagnan
800-327-8246
www.dartagnan.com

A variety of fine organic products, including:

Buffalo
Raised free of hormones and antibiotics. A delicious and nutritional meat.

Free Range Australian Lamb
Raised free of hormones and antibiotics.

Eberly Free Range Organic Chicken

Nuts, Nut Butters, and Seeds

Living Tree Community Foods
800-260-5534
www.livingtreecommunity.com

Organically grown nuts, seeds, and butters, including almonds (many varieties), macadamia nuts, pinenuts, pumpkin seeds, sunflower seeds, walnut quarters, raw almond butter, and raw cashew butter. The products are refrigerated until shipped.

Tree of Life
Tree of Life Creamy Cashew Butter
Tree of Life Organic Sesame Tahini
Tree of Life Organic Almond Butter—Creamy or Crunchy
Good sources of vitamins, essential fatty acids, minerals, and protein.

Oils

Omega Nutrition
Essential Balance Jr.
A proprietary mixture of five fresh-pressed oils, scientifically blended in the evolutionary 1:1 omega-3 to omega-6 ratio. Contains certified organic flax, sunflower, sesame, pumpkin, and borage oils. Also contains gamma-linolenic acid (GLA) and omega-6 fatty acids, which diabetics often cannot produce. Butterscotch flavored.

Flax Seed Oil
Unrefined and certified organic, grown without pesticides or artificial fertilizers, and processed using Omega's exclusive omegaflo® process.

Olive Oil
Made from unrefined, extra-virgin olives that are fresh-pressed and omegaflo® bottled.

Tree of Life®
High Lignan Flax Oil
Contains all the antioxidants of their original Organic Flax Oil plus high fiber lignans. Liquid form.

Poultry

Sheltons Poultry, Inc.
800-541-1844

Free-range chicken and turkey raised without antibiotics. Noted health expert Andrew Weil, M.D., cautions people to avoid eating poultry and meat raised with antibiotics, which have been linked to drug-resistant strains of disease-causing bacteria.

Seafood

Capilano Pacific
877-391-WILD (9453)
www.capilanopacific.com

Wildfish™
A wonderful source for wild-caught salmon. Most of the salmon available in restaurants and stores was farm-raised. Usually, this means it was raised on feed containing antibiotics and synthetic coloring. Wild-caught salmon ate natural food, plus has a high level of omega-3 fatty acids and much less fat than farm-raised salmon. It tastes better as well. Also available are halibut, tuna, and lox.

Special Drinks With Electrolytes

Moss Nutrition
Balance Electrolyte
For mothers to be and young mothers who work out and require electrolyte replacement. Unlike commercial drinks, this electrolyte solution has no added sugars or sweeteners.

Stevia

Wisdom of the Ancients®
800-899-9908
www.wisdomherbs.com

Natural sweetener made from whole leaf stevia *(Stevia rebaudiana Bertoni)*. A 6:1 concentrated extract. Available as concentrated tablets, liquid, and tea. Hundreds of scientific studies have been conducted of stevia's effectiveness as a nutritional support for the pancreas.

Teas (Green)

Try switching from coffee to green tea and enjoy the benefits of antioxidants and less caffeine. Actually, there is an amino acid in green tea *(Camellia sinensis)* that balances caffeine's effects and delivers a sense of relaxation. Also, as noted earlier in this book, too much caffeine can interfere with sleep, making mother and baby jittery.

Great Eastern Sun
800-334-5809
www.great-eastern-sun.com

Haiku® Organic Japanese Teas
Organic Original Sencha Green Tea: The finest grade of green leaf tea available, made from the tender young leaves of selected tea bushes, cut at the peak of their flavor, rolled, steamed, and briefly dried. Contains 100% Nagata Japanese organic Sencha green tea leaves and buds. Available in tea bags and bulk.

Organic Original Hojicha Roasted Green Tea: Lower in caffeine than Sencha, Hojicha has a subtle smoky and rich flavor that is quite different from that of Sencha. Contains 100% Nagata Japanese organic Hojicha roasted green tea leaves and stems. Available in tea bags and bulk.

Great Eastern Sun carries a full line of delicious organic classic teas and flavored tea blends including:

Organic Ceylon Highland: Nothing but 100% famed mountain-grown Sri Lankan leaf from the Thotulagalla and Green Fields Organic Estates goes into this smooth, full flavored tea. It's rich yet delicate taste can be enjoyed any time of day (especially in the morning!) and is delicious hot or iced. Contains organic Ceylon black tea.

Organic Darjeeling Thunder Bolt: Grown exclusively for One World® on the Makaibari Organic Estate on the pristine slopes of the Himalayan Mountains of northern India, this refined tea has a flavor so unique it has been called "the champagne of teas." Fragrant aroma and rich taste make it the finest of India's unblended teas.

Organic Zanzibar Orange Spice: Meticulously formulated, One World® Organic Orange Spice is a superb combination of organic cut black teas flavored with organic orange peel, organic cloves, organic cinnamon, and organic orange oil.

Triple Leaf Tea, Inc.
800-552-7448
www.tripleleaf-tea.com

http://www.tripleleaf-tea.com
maryanne@tripleleaf-tea.com

Effective, authentic, traditional Chinese green, naturally decaffeinated green, medicinal, and diet teas, made with authentic Chinese herbs and traditional herbal formulas, packaged in convenient tea bag form. All teas are GMO-free.

Decaf Green Tea
Decaf Green Tea Blends
Made using a natural solvent-free carbon dioxide decaffeination process that researchers have found maintains almost all of green tea's beneficial antioxidants, including EGCG, while leaving no chemical residue. Two other decaffeination methods use either a chemical solvent, ethyl acetate, which researchers have found to remove much of the antioxidants, or water, which also is likely to lose the antioxidants, since they are extremely water-soluble.

If you drink a lot of tea and don't want the caffeine, this is the ideal tea to use.

Jasmine Green Tea
Made from jasmine flowers combined with green tea, creating a delicious aromatic tea. Jasmine was traditionally used for its calming, relaxing, and warming properties, for brightening the mood, and as a soothing digestive tea.

Triple Leaf Tea, Inc., also carries a delicious and spicy 100% ginger root tea, and 100% American ginseng root tea, to support balance, health, and well-being.

Tree of Life®
www.treeoflife.com
There are many fine health-food stores all over the country that carry top-notch products. Many stores are supplied by an excellent company known as Tree of Life, a distributor of high quality natural foods at moderate prices. When shopping at health-food stores, you can ask for Tree of Life products. If a store doesn't carry a particular product, ask to have it ordered.

Tree of Life Frozen Organic Vegetables
Certified organically grown. Broccoli, corn, green peas, spinach.

Tree of Life Frozen Organic Fruit
Loaded with nutrients without any added chemicals. They are often difficult to obtain. Strawberries, blueberries, raspberries.

Tree of Life Frozen Smoothie Makers
Fresh-frozen chunks of 100% organic fruit. Ideal for jucing. Banana, raspberry strawberry.

Tree of Life Pasta Sauce
Original and salt-free. In glass jars. This organic pasta sauce is made from vine-ripened, specially selected premium tomatoes that are grown for their sweetness and flavor.

Tree of Life Organic Tamari and Shoyu
Made from organic soybeans and wheat. Excellent for steamed vegetables and fish. Shoyu, wheat-free tamari.

Natural Detoxification and Cleansing

When taking charge of your health, your child's health, or your unborn child's health, it is very important to avoid toxins in the food you eat, the water you drink, the air you breathe, and virtually all the products you use, from shampoos and toothpaste to cleansers and cosmetics. The companies listed here offer the highest quality products. If you cannot find their products at your local health food store, please contact these companies directly for the store nearest you.

Dental Products

Woodstock Natural Products, Inc.
800-615-6895

The Natural Dentist™
There is a holistic connection between the health of your teeth and gums, and your whole body. This is especially true for diabetics, who need to be vigilant about their teeth and gums because they have a tendency to develop periodontal disease. Woodstock Natural Products are formulated by a holistic dentist and contain soothing and healing herbs, with no alcohol, sugar, or harsh chemicals. These products have been clinically proven to kill germs that cause gum disease. In a study published in the *Journal of Clinical Dentistry* in 1998, researchers at the New York University College of Dentistry in New York City found that The Natural Dentist toothpaste removed plauqe more effectively than the leading commercial brand. The same group also found that The Natural Dentist mouth rinse killed more germs than the leading commercial brand.
Toothpaste: mint, cinnamon, and fluoride-free mint.
Mouth rinse: mint, cinnamon, and cherry.

Desert Essence®
888-476-8647
www.desertessence.com

Oral Care Collection
A complete line of antiseptic and cleansing oral care products using tea tree oil for deep cleaning and disinfecting of teeth and gums. All products are animal and eco-friendly, and made without artificial colors, sweeteners, or harsh abrasives.

Tea Tree Oil Dental Floss: Creates a germ-free mouth and cleans between the teeth.
Tea Tree Oil Dental Tape: Provides the same benefits as floss with a wider ribbon.
Tea Tree Oil Dental Pics: Cleans between the teeth with antiseptic power.
Tea Tree Oil Breath Freshener: Contains natural and organic essental oils.

N.E.E.D.S. (Mail Order)
800-634-1380
www.needs.com

An excellent resource for top-notch environmental products, including the following:

Aireox Air Purifier (Model 45): Removes mold spores, pollen dust, formaldehyde, and more.

Aireox Car Air Purifier (Model 22): An unusual purifier for the car.

Allens Naturally: A full line of toxin-free household cleansers, including dishwashing and laundry detergents and all-purpose cleaners.

Water Filters
N.E.E.D.S. carries a variety of high-quality water filters.

Elite Shower Filter and Massager: For removing chlorine, heavy metals, and bacteria.

Natural Cosmetics

Carlson®
E-Gem® Oil Drops
Each drop contains 10 IU of natural vitamin E; $\frac{1}{2}$ oz contains 5,000 IU of vitamin E. Apply externally to aid and soften skin.

E-Gem® Organic Shampoo
Formulated with natural vitamin E, vitamins A and D, panthenol, and protein.

Garden Fresh Soap
100% vegetarian. Contains aloe vera, avocado, cucumber, carrot oil, olive oil, and other ingredients.

Jason Natural Costmetics
800-JASON-05
www.jason-natural.com
Chamomile Liquid Satin Soap™ with Pump
Natural Sea Kelp Shampoo

INDEX